Pelvic Floor Recovery

Physiotherapy for
Gynaecological and Colorectal Repair Surgery

(4th Edition)

Sue Croft
Physiotherapist
www.suecroftphysiotherapist.com.au

*This book is dedicated to my wonderful family, my beautiful staff
and my fantastic patients!*

About the Author

Sue Croft *is a physiotherapist in private practice with a special interest in continence, pelvic health and pelvic pain. Sue graduated from the University of Queensland with a Bachelor of Physiotherapy in 1977 and since 1989 has worked in women's health and continence promotion for women, men and children. Sue is currently a registered physiotherapist, a member of the Australian Physiotherapy Association, the National Women's, Men's and Pelvic Health Physiotherapy Group, the International Continence Society, IUGA and a Committee member of the Queensland Branch of the Continence Foundation of Australia.*

Pelvic Floor Recovery

Physiotherapy for Gynaecological and Colorectal Repair Surgery
by Sue Croft. 4th Edition.

Copyright© Sue Croft 2018
www.pelvicfloorrecovery.com
Illustrations by Bob Croft
Cover original painting by Katie Martel

ISBN 9780648264408

A catalogue record for this book is available from the National Library of Australia

Foreword

by Dr Hannah Krause AO MBBS FRANZCOG CU MPhil

It is with pleasure that I write this foreword to encourage women to actively participate in their own pelvic floor recovery and to congratulate Sue on publishing the 4th edition of *Pelvic Floor Recovery*. This edition has been expanded with advice for those undergoing colorectal surgery and has been retitled *Pelvic Floor Recovery - Physiotherapy for Gynaecological and Colorectal Repair Surgery*.

Sue's earlier editions have been read and studied by countless women, including many of my own patients, since first published in 2011. *Pelvic Floor Recovery* is an informative and a very practical handbook which guides women in understanding their diagnosis of pelvic floor dysfunction and gives advice on pelvic floor rehabilitation. Pre and post-operative physiotherapy management and an emphasis on how to protect the pelvic floor during daily activities and exercise are important concepts to help minimize the progression and recurrence of pelvic floor problems.

As a urogynaecologist, I advocate a team approach to optimize the outcomes of women suffering with pelvic floor dysfunction. I do recommend all women consult with a pelvic floor physiotherapist to instruct them on pelvic floor rehabilitation and to actively pursue the positive conservative management options contained in Sue's book.

This 4th edition includes additional information and an update on recent research on prolapse and also includes Sue's innovative acronym *'PIPES'* as an assessment tool in pelvic floor dysfunction. I anticipate that this updated version of *Pelvic Floor Recovery* will continue to inform, educate and encourage women to improve their pelvic floor function and quality of life.

*Sue would like to acknowledge **Dr Hannah Krause AO** who has kindly written the foreword for this book. Dr Krause is a subspecialist in urogynaecology working in Brisbane. Dr Krause also teaches medical students and registrars, and lectures other health care professionals in Australia and overseas, in topics of urogynaecology. She has published research in peer-review journals and is actively involved in research with women suffering pelvic floor dysfunction.*

*She frequently travels to parts of Africa and Asia as a medical volunteer to treat women with childbirth injuries including obstetric fistulae and severe pelvic organ prolapse and to train and upskill local practitioners. **Donations** to support the invaluable work Dr Hannah Krause undertakes in Africa and Asia can be made through an organization called HADA (**www.hada.org.au, Donations, Medical Training in Africa and Asia (AFR-010)**. Sue is grateful to Hannah for her kind words.*

Contents

Contents

Introduction

'Let's make sure your first op is your best op and hopefully your last op.'

This is a patient-directed book which I first published in 2011 at the request of numerous patients who wanted more detailed information to help them navigate the challenging path of urogenital surgery. Although the first three editions of this book were more directed towards gynaecological surgery, over the years many patients undergoing colorectal surgery also found those editions helpful. It is for this reason that I have included more information specific to colorectal surgery in this edition.

Gynaecological surgery is undertaken when women for different reasons require a hysterectomy or need repair surgery for the management of urinary incontinence or pelvic organ prolapse. Urinary incontinence (UI) is prevalent – one in three women will suffer with incontinence in their lifetime[1] and while conservative treatment from a physiotherapist has impressive results[2,3,4] some women will require a surgical intervention to get them dry. However, there have been issues with some of the continence surgery devices and at the time of writing this edition, some of the implants used in urinary incontinence surgery have been withdrawn because of complications. Therefore, the conservative management strategies in this book have even more relevance.

The research also tells us that up to 50% of women who have had a vaginal delivery will suffer from prolapse in their lifetime, so the potential for repair surgery is significant if conservative measures have failed.[5] 10% to 20% of women with prolapse will undergo surgery in their lifetime and up to 30% of those women will need to undergo a further repair due to recurrence of the prolapse.[6][7] Undertaking lifelong preventative strategies such as those contained in this book will hopefully empower you to look after your surgery.

Colorectal repair surgery is undertaken for women (and men) when they have conditions such as rectal prolapse, intussusception, faecal incontinence, haemorrhoids and anal fissures. Similarly colorectal repair surgery can fail if changes are not made to the technique that patients employ to defaecate. Straining at stool and bowel dysfunction is common and due to the personal nature of the problem is often under-reported and not openly discussed even with doctors. Understanding about the correct dynamics of passing a bowel motion is critical post-colorectal surgery to ensure there is no recurrence of the initial problem.

Throughout this book I refer to research which shows that the conservative management of pelvic floor dysfunction by a physiotherapist with a special interest in pelvic health, should be the first line of treatment.[8] For this reason this book has considerable information on normal and abnormal bladder and bowel function, pelvic floor activation and strengthening, pelvic organ prolapse and the preventative treatment strategies. Even if you identify that your problem is only stress incontinence or prolapse, you should read the whole book to help prevent other longer term bladder and bowel dysfunction which can happen by continuing incorrect habits.

However, there are situations when conservative measures are not always fully successful and surgery is necessary. In our time-poor society there is a mantra of *'let's do it and do it quick'*! However, where repair operations are concerned, a measured carefully planned approach with excellent preparation can save distress and promote a better outcome for the patient and surgeon.

Understanding the process of surgery and having some basic understanding of terminology and procedure will give confidence to the patient during their hospital stay and therefore improve the quality of the experience. I believe this book will provide strategies to give you the best chance of a successful long-term outcome following your gynaecological or colorectal repair surgery.

Many simple daily tasks undertaken such as housework, shopping and minding young children can present you with a situation post-operatively where you are placing too much strain on your surgery - at a time before maximal fibrosis of the repair has occurred at around 12 weeks when collagen will reach 80% of its tensile strength.[9] This useful scar tissue assists in the stabilising of your repair operation.

More and more women of all ages are aware of the health benefits of maintaining a regular cardiovascular exercise and strength training for staving off the debilitating consequences of osteoporosis, obesity and mental health decline. However if after surgery you return to exercise too early or if you overload the strength of *your* pelvic floor muscles, your repair may be compromised and there can be recurrence of the incontinence and prolapse problems. I hope this book will further enhance your chance of a positive outcome and encourage you to embark on an exercise program after your operation.

In this book there is a chapter on persistent pelvic pain and an outline of treatment strategies for pain such as abdominal and pelvic floor muscle relaxation, breath awareness exercises and the use of vaginal dilators should they be necessary.

There is a comprehensive outline of physiotherapy strategies to be undertaken before and after your repair surgery, with sections on *'pelvic floor friendly'* abdominal exercises, your return to general exercise and sport, sexual function, resuming work and travel advice.

Empowering women with information about normal bladder and bowel function will not only assist in a more successful post-operative outcome, but will also ensure dissemination of correct science about the bladder, bowel and prolapse to their children, grandchildren, family, friends and neighbours. This book allows women to find answers to embarrassing questions by covering the taboo subjects of bowels and sex. It also provides links to relevant websites and further reading, but importantly, it will give assurance that their doctor can provide them with more detailed information - *if they just ask them the question!*

The strategies outlined in this book are simple, preventative measures designed to pre-operatively strengthen the pelvic floor muscles and to ensure that you have a comfortable, stress-free stay in hospital and return post-operatively to home, work and exercise armed with evidence-based information. These strategies will hopefully contribute towards a good long-term outcome following your surgery. Read the book thoroughly before and after your operation implementing as much of the book as you can. Revisit the book once each year to ensure that you are maintaining good pelvic floor health and well-being for the rest of your life.

My most important goal is to enhance your
'Pelvic Floor Recovery'.

Sue Croft

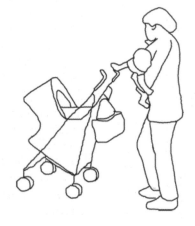

Understanding pelvic floor dysfunction

Managing pelvic floor dysfunction is a complex and important area in preventative medicine. Society places enormous significance on being dry and toilet trained by early age. A Deloitte Access Economics project (2011), commissioned by the Continence Foundation of Australia, the peak body in Australia and a world leader in continence promotion, has shown the prevalence of incontinence in Australia is approximately 4.2 million men, women and children (over the age of 15 years) which will increase significantly in future years due to the burgeoning ageing population. The financial burden to the national economy through loss of productivity (people with incontinence and their carers are less likely to work) and due to the cost of continence aids was approximately $40 billion per annum back when this extensive study was done.[1] **Incontinence is a huge and expensive problem**.

When bladder and bowel systems fail, damage occurs to self-esteem and self-worth, whether it be a young woman who is unable to play sport without leaking after a vaginal delivery; a lady who is post-menopausal and loses control of her bladder when she turns on a tap; a man following prostate surgery, who for the first time in his life is confronted with pads to deal with the indignity of leaking or, more relevant to this text, a woman whose gynaecological or colorectal repair surgery may have had a less than favorable outcome.

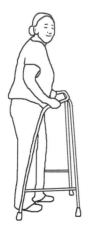

The following information on bladder and bowel problems should be *revisited regularly* to ensure ongoing maintenance of your bladder, bowel and your pelvic floor function. The good bladder and bowel recommendations that follow should be *lifelong* habits which, if adopted, will optimize better function in this area. Many elderly men and women are placed in nursing homes, not necessarily only because of dementia or physical impairment, but rather because of the impact of urinary and faecal incontinence on their carers. Simple preventative measures adopted early and maintained throughout your life will hopefully prevent the insidious, progressive nature of many types of pelvic floor dysfunction.

The pelvic floor muscles

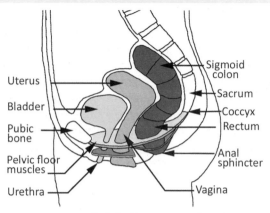

Fig 1. **Pelvic floor muscles**
(Adapted from C. Maher & S. Francis)

Treating the whole pelvis

"As we learn more about the natural function and causes of dysfunction of the female pelvis, we are beginning to see that the parts can no longer be regarded in isolation. Rather, the components must be thought of in relation to the whole pelvis and therefore the whole patient." Dr Michael P. Aronson
American Journal 'Obstetrics and Gynaecology' 1994

Many years ago, this quote started my journey towards understanding that managing incontinence and other forms of pelvic floor dysfunction was not only about the pelvic floor muscles. It became apparent that our system needs to be finely tuned and well-coordinated. We need to understand the cross-talk between the bladder and bowel; to acknowledge the failure of connective tissue and of ligament support and the potential for muscle trauma due to childbirth; and know about the interaction of the pelvic floor muscles, the abdominal muscles and the diaphragm which work closely together to provide continence control, pelvic organ support and urinary and faecal elimination for an individual.

Every day women have to deal with loads and forces that require a finely tuned coordination of muscles, ligamentous support and of the nervous system, in order to provide continence control and internal organ support. These mechanisms may be compromised due to pregnancy, childbirth and a myriad of other health problems and challenged by the jobs and activities required in any given day. Understanding about the integrated anatomy of the components of this highly coordinated system will enhance the function of the bladder, bowel and pelvic floor.

The pelvic floor muscles *(Fig 1)* sit at the base of our body and provide the floor of our pelvis. They support the bladder, uterus and rectum and assist with effective function of those organs. There are two layers of muscles – the superficial layers compress the entrance of the vagina and anus and are important sexual muscles and assist with gas and faecal control. The deeper layers (the levator ani muscles) contribute to continence control, increased sexual awareness and pelvic organ support helping to prevent prolapse. They are striated muscles, which means they are under your voluntary control and as such can be exercised to strengthen them.

What does a well-activated pelvic floor do?

- It adds to the closing force for the bladder and back passage, preventing leakage of urine, gas and faeces.

- Research tells us that between 60% to 80% of women with stress urinary incontinence can be improved and cured with *pelvic floor muscle training (PFMT)*[2,3,4] and timely recruitment of the muscles (known as 'the knack') with increased intra-abdominal pressure (e.g. cough, sneeze, jump)[10].

- It should relax to allow easy and complete emptying of the bladder and if recruited again after completion of urination can prevent a dribble after voiding (called a post-micturition dribble).

- It should relax to allow complete evacuation of the bowel, while still providing the necessary support and resistance to allow effective defaecation.

- It assists with support of the internal organs of the pelvis - the bladder, vagina and rectum. The more intact the muscles are following a vaginal delivery, the less the likelihood of prolapse.

- It increases the tone within the vaginal walls and increases sexual awareness. It needs to be able to relax to have pleasurable pain-free sex.

- It relaxes and significantly stretches during a vaginal delivery.

- It works in a coordinated way with the abdominal muscles and your breathing (the diaphragm).

9

How do you strengthen the pelvic floor?

Pelvic floor muscle training (PFMT)

- Initially start in the lying position (to take weight off the muscles). Keep your spine neutral – neither arched or flattened. Start by establishing low slow breathing. Do not puff up your chest. Keep your shoulders relaxed and feel the gentle rise and fall of the abdominal wall as you breathe.

- Draw the muscles *gently* in and up around the urethra, vagina and anus (as if you are stopping the flow of urine and/or holding in wind) while you continue to breathe. Contracting the muscles gently is important when first learning how to correctly activate the muscles. The action you should feel is **lift and squeeze pressure.** You should not feel pressure pushing down (called bearing down). This is the wrong action. If you feel pushing down then stop attempting to do the pelvic floor contractions.

- It is important to seek help from a pelvic health physiotherapist if there is any doubt about how to contract the muscles correctly. Research shows that around 30% of women perform their pelvic floor muscle contractions wrongly when merely following a leaflet or book.[11] If you are bearing down instead of getting lift and squeeze, this may make your incontinence and prolapse worse.

- Research has shown also that PFMT is significantly more effective if performed in a supervised setting such as with a physiotherapist.[12,13]

- If you cannot feel the sensation of lift, then you can improve your biofeedback (messages back to your brain) by inserting your finger into the vagina to feel if the muscles are lifting and squeezing. (If you do this, place your finger directly on the pelvic floor muscles on both the right and left side to feel them working).

- *Keep breathing* as you hold the contraction. At the same time place your fingers on the pubic hair line and you may feel your *lower* abdomen around your pubic hair line gently tension, drawing away from your fingers. Do not flare your ribs or try too hard; do not suck your belly button to your spine.

Remember:
"Start where you are. Use what you have. Do what you can."

Arthur Ashe, American social activist and champion tennis player.

- To voluntarily activate striated muscles (ones you can exercise) we have to have the appropriate brain 'conceptualization' of that particular movement.[11] You have never *'seen'* your pelvic floor muscles like you have *'seen'* your biceps muscle. Utilizing our most powerful organ in our body - *the brain* - to visualize the correct action (lift and squeeze) of the pelvic floor is also very useful, so viewing an image of where the muscles are located can also help. See the image of the inside of a pelvis below and look at those muscles as you attempt to contract them. Imagine them drawing up and in.

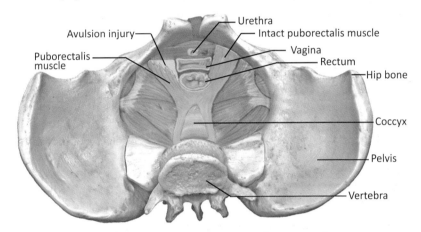

Urethra
Avulsion injury
Intact puborectalis muscle
Puborectalis muscle
Vagina
Rectum
Hip bone
Coccyx
Pelvis
Vertebra

Fig 2. **Top view of the pelvic floor muscles**
It can help to use this image of the pelvic floor
muscles to visualize the muscles you are trying to
contract when doing your muscle training.
Copyright© Sue Croft 2018

- To start with, only hold your pelvic floor contraction for a few seconds; then build up gradually to a *10 to 15 second hold* and ultimately longer while **continuing to breathe**. Initially practise *3 to 5 at a time* to avoid fatigue of the muscles and so you can hold your 'form'.

- Remember many women following childbirth may have significant nerve or muscle damage (levator avulsion - *page 16*)[14] and may have very weak pelvic floor muscles. Even if there is significant damage to the muscles, it is very important to try to exercise the remaining fibres of the muscles.

- A *well-coordinated, long endurance muscle* is, for some women, as important as a *strong* muscle especially if there is levator avulsion.

- Remember, if holding your abdominal muscles and pelvic floor muscles constantly 'on', then doing more pelvic floor muscle contractions may cause pelvic pain. *Always relax your pelvic floor muscles and tummy muscles after a series of exercises.*

- If you have normal muscle activation, then because the pelvic floor muscles are striated (voluntary) muscles, when you perform exercise repetitions of these muscles, they can bulk up and strengthen. Turning these stronger muscles on at the right time *('the knack')*[10] can improve stress urinary incontinence

- When working out your exercise program, if we look at general exercise science, healthy voluntary muscle can increase its strength by up to 30% after an intensive 8 to 12 week program of muscle strengthening.[11]

- When working out your exercise program, when we look at general exercise science, for strength training we need to do *5 to 10 contractions 3 times per day.*[11] It is better to do fewer muscle exercises that are of a high quality than do 300 quick short ones when you may lose form, fatigue or even start bearing down. Many women over the years have been told to do 300 Kegel exercises a day (named after Dr Kegel who is attributed with first teaching women about pelvic floor muscles). Fortunately, this number is not necessary.

- Research in Norway has found that after an intensive pelvic floor muscle training program, the thickness of the pelvic floor muscles can result in a decrease in the internal gap (the levator hiatus) and lifting of the pelvic organs.[15,16]

If you aim to do 5 to 10 contractions, 3 times per day (fairly intensively) as long as there is some healthy muscle present, after 8 to 12 weeks you should notice an improvement in strength of your pelvic floor muscles.

- Lifetime adherence to exercising the pelvic floor is important, as a 5% to 10% loss of muscle strength per week has been shown after ceasing your PFMT (exercises) and this is worse in older age groups (65 to 75 years) compared to younger (20 to 30 years).[17]

- We know from research that long term compliance with any pelvic floor exercise program is a major problem for patients and as PFMT is one of the major components of your treatment program for urinary incontinence, faecal incontinence and prolapse management, it is important to schedule regular exercises and incorporate PFMT into any general exercise you do. However, studies seem to indicate that while the *intensity* of the exercise should be maintained, the frequency and number of exercises can reduce after the initial 12 week period to fewer exercises, one to two days a week to maintain strength gains or slow strength losses.[17]

- After the early training phase, it is then important to integrate the pelvic floor contractions into your every day movements and exercises *(Chapter 11)*. Contracting maximally for high pressure activities (cough and sneeze) and less intensively for lower pressure activities becomes easier as you incorporate them in your daily life.
- Other forms of treatment that may be offered for strengthening pelvic floor muscles may include biofeedback devices, vaginal weighted cones, electrical stimulation and muscle vibration. See the link in *Appendix 1* to a very reputable online pelvic health site where pelvic health equipment can be purchased for home use or under the supervision of your physiotherapist.
- There are also many smart phone apps to assist you with remembering to do your pelvic floor muscle training.
- The biggest barrier to your improvement with your pelvic floor dysfunction is a lack of compliance with your program. Doing some regular work with your PF muscles is going to maximize your chances of less problems as you age.

The dos and don'ts of correctly contracting your pelvic floor muscles <u>when first learning them</u>:

- *Do not use your inner thigh muscles.*
- *Do not tilt your pelvis.*
- *Do not clench your buttocks.*
- *Do not strongly contract your abdominal muscles.*
- *Do not hold your breath.*
- *Do not bear down.*
- *Do not flare your ribs*
- *Yes, you should feel lift and squeeze of the pelvic floor.*
- *Yes, your lower tummy may draw gently in.*
- *Yes, initially gentle is better than trying too hard to ensure the correct activation.*
- *Yes, when you are sure you have the correct activation, you can add some maximal contractions.*
- *Yes, always remember to let go and relax your pelvic floor muscles after exercising them.*

- *Stand* with your legs apart and toes turned in and then try a pelvic floor contraction. This position will help you minimize overflow into the adductor (inner thigh) muscles and assist in better sensation of lift of the pelvic floor. It is important to train your muscles in this more difficult *'loaded'* position *(Fig 3)*.

- *Sit tall* and upright away from the back of your chair with your legs slightly apart and maintaining your lumbar curve. Feel your perineum (urethral/vaginal area) resting on the seat. Try to draw in and lift your pelvic floor up off the firm seat. Placing your hand there will also give you good feedback *(Fig 4)*.

- *Lean forward on the chair* to feel more awareness around the anal sphincter and imagine you have a sharp thing such as a pin sitting at the anus (ouch!). Try and draw your anus away from that sharp thing. **Use your brain** to visualize these actions at the anus and it may help gain a better response in the muscles *(Fig 5 on page 17)*.

- *Lie on your tummy* if you are able. (If you are breast feeding, overweight or older you may find this position difficult). Start by breathing low and slow and then try to draw in around the urethra, vagina and anus. In this position you will often feel a better peri-urethral (around the urethra) sensation of lift.

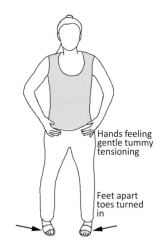

Hands feeling gentle tummy tensioning

Feet apart toes turned in

- If you feel uncomfortable lying on your tummy then try the exercise in standing, leaning forwards onto a bench with your feet 45 cm (18 inches) away from the bench to do the exercises *(Fig 8 on page 22)*. You need good balance to try this exercise so always make sure you are safe when attempting this leaning exercise.

*Fig 3. **Pelvic floor exercises in standing position***
© Sue Croft 2018

How do you know if you are doing the right exercise?

- *Feeling for lift*: Place your hand firmly under your perineum (the part resting on the chair between your legs) as you sit up tall in a chair. As you draw up the pelvic floor muscles, feel your perineum gently lift up from your hand. If you feel a sense of bulging down, *stop* doing the exercise. This is called *'bearing down'*. Always do some specific anal sphincter exercises as well.

- *Change in Symptoms*: Your problems of leakage or lack of control should begin to improve if you are doing the correct program. If there is no improvement, your program needs to be reviewed by a pelvic health physiotherapist. If symptoms become worse, **stop** doing your pelvic floor muscle exercises and make a review appointment with your physiotherapist.

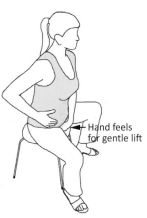

Hand feels for gentle lift

- *Stopping your urine mid-stream:* During urination, try to slow or stop the flow by drawing on your pelvic floor muscles. (*Do not* try this when your bladder is very full. *Do not* do this if you have any retention problems with your bladder when voiding. *Repeat only once a month* as a test). However this is *not* a definitive test of strength.

Fig 4. **Pelvic floor exercises in sitting position**
© Sue Croft 2018

- *Improved sensory awareness*: The pelvic floor muscles often respond very well to small amounts of input, so you will often become more aware of your pelvic floor muscles and feel improvement quite quickly, unless you have had significant muscle trauma such as levator avulsion *(page 16)*. If you are sexually active, you may often feel better awareness during intercourse as your muscles get stronger.

Important:
If you feel your pelvic floor pushing down when you attempt a pelvic floor contraction, stop exercising and seek help with a pelvic health physiotherapist who can do an internal examination and teach you the correct action.

What affects strength of the pelvic floor muscles?

Sometimes vaginal deliveries can cause structural damage to the pelvic floor muscles by directly tearing the muscles partially or completely from their attachment on the pelvis (called *levator avulsion*) or can compress or traction the nerves that innervate the muscles causing temporary or permanent injury.

What is Levator Avulsion?

The levator ani muscles (the muscles of the pelvic floor) form the levator hiatus which is the internal space of the vagina containing the urethra to the front, the vagina centrally, and the ano-rectum at the back.[18] It is crucial in supporting your internal pelvic organs and the maintenance of both the urinary and faecal continence mechanism. The levator hiatus represents the largest portal (opening) in the human body.[18]

Avulsion injuries are when there is a disconnection of the muscle from its insertion on the bony parts of the pelvis due to vaginal delivery and are known to occur in up to 20% of women who have had babies.[18] The research tells us that there is an increased risk of prolapse due to avulsion following vaginal deliveries. As the muscles have pulled off the bone, the levator hiatus (gap in the vagina) is wider. There is likely to be ballooning of the vagina and therefore a clear opportunity for the internal organs to relax or prolapse downwards with increases in intra-abdominal pressure such as with repetitive coughing and sneezing, heavy lifting and other activities of daily living. Significant levator avulsion increases the risk of anterior (front) wall or uterine prolapse by up to three times.[19] See *Fig 2, page 11*.

An analogy to make the concept of how levator avulsion weakens the pelvic floor muscles easier to understand is if half of your deltoid (shoulder) muscle was partially torn from its attachment, then it would be difficult to lift your arm out to the side Similarly, if you have significant unilateral (one sided) or bilateral avulsion (both sides) of the pelvic floor muscles due to a vaginal delivery, then you may be trying very hard with your pelvic floor exercises (PFMT) but not feel any improvement in strength. This is because the muscles are no longer attached completely to the pelvis and are unable to build up strength through repetition training.

The avulsion injuries vary from woman to woman and there is very often some fibres still attached and it is important to continue to do pelvic floor exercises to maximize the potential of any remaining muscle. Levator avulsion is strongly associated with: the age of the mother, (more than triples during the reproductive years from below 15% when the mother is aged 20 years, to over

50% at when aged 40 years)[20]; long second stage of labour; posterior presentation of the baby; baby's weight over 4kg and the use of forceps[21] but can also happen in vaginal deliveries with no instruments. There can also be irreversible over-stretching of the levator gap in more than 25% of women who have had vaginal deliveries, often due to micro-trauma of the muscles which contributes to the looseness of the vaginal walls often experienced by women during exercise and intercourse.[21] A simple measurement called **GH+PB valsalva** can be performed by your pelvic health physiotherapist to help predict your risk of prolapse following a vaginal delivery.[20] It measures the distance halfway through the urethra to half-way through the anal sphincter on maximum valsalva - which is when you push down into your vagina like you are pushing a baby out, holding for 6 seconds. A measurement less than 7cm is normal, greater than 8.5cm may indicate the presence of levator avulsion and increased vaginal distensibility. (See *page 106* for full values)

Nerve damage

Vaginal deliveries can also cause temporary or permanent neurogenic (nerve) changes.[11] This occurs via *compression* to the nerves or their blood supply or via *traction* (over-stretch) of the nerves leading to temporary or permanent damage. There can be motor (movement) damage causing weakness of the muscles and sensory denervation (awareness of sensation to the area) affecting the ability of the woman to feel the muscles moving. As there is sometimes significant nerve damage, this can even affect the continuous (motor) activity in the sphincter muscles at rest and when you go to sleep. There can be some gradual improvement to nerve function over time if there is only partial damage to the nerves. Electrical stimulation of the muscles via an E-stim machine, which can be purchased for home use, can be taught to you by your physiotherapist.

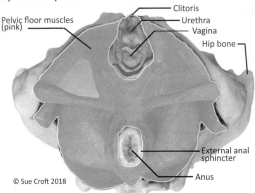

Clitoris
Pelvic floor muscles (pink)
Urethra
Vagina
Hip bone
External anal sphincter
Anus
© Sue Croft 2018

*Fig 5. **Under view of the pelvic floor muscles***

It can help to use this image of the pelvic floor muscles to visualize the muscles you are trying to contract when you are muscle training.

The interaction of the abdominal and pelvic floor muscles

The pelvic floor muscles work intimately with the abdominal muscles. Understanding this interaction *may* be useful for improving bladder and bowel function, especially when trying to empty your bladder or bowel. It is virtually impossible to contract your pelvic floor muscles without contracting your abdominal muscles. The deepest or fourth layer of the abdominal muscles, the *transversus abdominis (TA)*, assists the pelvic floor muscles with urethral closing pressure and through co-contraction helps to activate the pelvic floor. Drawing in your lower abdomen gently, may *sometimes* facilitate an enhanced pelvic floor contraction, *but does not replace the important role of pelvic floor muscle training.* It is important to be sure you are not getting downward movement into the vagina when attempting abdominal muscle contractions.

When attempting to find the TA, it is important to continue to breathe gently, being careful to avoid rib flaring and apical chest breathing (up high in your chest). However some women may excessively recruit their abdominal muscles and cause bearing down into their vagina - so being assessed with an internal examination by a physiotherapist is the best way to ensure this is not happening. Understanding this interaction is vital if you have pelvic pain, voiding dysfunction or defaecation difficulties, as it is important to *relax your abdomen* to help relax your pelvic floor muscles which can interfere with evacuation and increase pain with intercourse.

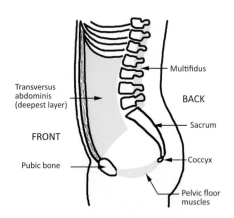

*Fig 6. **Abdominal muscles and the pelvic floor***
© Sue Croft 2018

How do I activate the deep abdominal muscles?

Start by lying flat on a bed, with your knees drawn up. To help you find the correct muscles, it can help if you imagine that you are putting on a tight pair of jeans. Visualize pulling up the zipper on the jeans and that it is pinching your skin or pubic hairs. So to avoid getting 'pinched', draw in at that pubic hairline *gently*. Continue to breathe in and out gently, while drawing in your low tummy. You may then feel your pelvic floor and anus draw in as well. *This is what you need to feel!*

Caution: If you feel a bulge at your low tummy (instead of a gentle tensioning or in-drawing) or pressure pushing down at the perineal region (around your vagina and anus) then you *must stop* and just concentrate on the pelvic floor muscle contractions. If you feel it sounds too complicated then concentrate on learning to do a pelvic floor contraction and stop trying to learn the TA contractions. You can seek help from a pelvic health physiotherapist. If you live in rural areas where you may not have access to such a specialized therapist, then a physiotherapist who has a real time ultrasound machine may be able to teach you the correct action of the pelvic floor muscles. (See *Appendix 1* to source a physiotherapist in your area through the APA website).

Are all abdominal strengthening muscles exercises good for my pelvic floor?

Sit-ups, full planks or double leg lifts increase your intra-abdominal pressure causing downward movement of the pelvic floor.[22] These types of exercises are best avoided if you have sustained significant damage to the muscles with a vaginal delivery; had gynaecological or colorectal repair surgery as they may cause pelvic organ prolapse; or if you have pelvic pain which may mean tightening these muscles more, could increase your pelvic pain. These types of movements may be a part of your pilates, yoga or aerobic classes at the gym and may need to be modified. If you have prolapse or a weak pelvic floor, remember to perform single leg lifts while protecting your pelvic floor by engaging the muscles (bracing/'the knack' see page 21) and avoid coming straight up into sitting from lying. 'Pelvic floor friendly' abdominal exercises are listed in chapter 11. Always do some quiet breathing and relax your tummy and pelvic floor after a session of exercising.

If you are sure you don't have pelvic floor dysfunction then sit-ups, full planks or double leg lifts are fine for you to do.

Role of the diaphragm and breath awareness

Get in touch with your body

The way you breathe has an important effect on the pelvic floor. In quiet inspiration, the diaphragm moves down and the abdominal wall moves forward. So, if you try too hard and precede a pelvic floor contraction with a big breath in, then your diaphragm pushes down and increases descent of the abdominal contents onto your internal organs and pelvic floor.

In quiet expiration, the diaphragm moves back up and the abdominal wall moves back to the original position. The pelvic floor muscles are active constantly but change length with breathing. They lengthen with inspiration and shorten with expiration. So, establishing a good breathing pattern is an important part of an effective pelvic floor and deep abdominal muscle training program.

Becoming aware of your breathing

Start learning about relaxed breathing in sitting as this stops the abdominal contents pushing the diaphragm up compared to lying. Keep your breathing low and slow. If you look at a mirror you can then ensure you are not *'puffing'* your chest up or *'flaring'* your ribs out which are often indicative of learning a poor pattern of breathing. As you become better with your breath awareness then you can practise in semi-reclining and then lying. If you hold your breath as you try to improve the endurance of your pelvic floor muscle contractions, you will cause descent of the bladder neck and pelvic organs. Remember to breathe on exertion (such as lifting). *Do not hold your breath!*

If you suffer a chronic respiratory condition such as hay fever, asthma, bronchitis, bronchiectasis, cystic fibrosis or chronic obstructive pulmonary disease (COPD) often known as emphysema, then there is an increased likelihood of pelvic floor dysfunction such as incontinence and prolapse. The pressure generated by a cough is extremely high, so including breath awareness practice, relaxation therapy and effective gentle recruitment of the pelvic floor muscles prior to coughing is critical ('the knack'/bracing *page 21*).

It is useful to practise and train bracing with coughing or blowing your nose, to develop these skills. Women can have a large abdominal muscle stretch or separation (rectus diastasis) following pregnancy and/or a weakened pelvic floor, which could result in a weak, ineffective cough and cause them to have difficulty clearing secretions if they have a respiratory condition.

Avoid breath holding– just keep breathing!

What is important? Bracing ('the knack')

If you search the internet for the meaning of the word *'bracing'*, a number of definitions pop up.[23]

- *To prepare for use.*
- *To get ready.*
- *A structural member used to stiffen a framework.*
- *A system of braces used to strengthen or support.*

It is with this in mind that I use the word *'bracing'* to teach my patients the importance of recruiting the correct muscles prior to increases in intra-abdominal pressure (IAP) with activities. Women have often read in magazines about the importance of doing regular pelvic floor exercises and yet by *only* doing those exercises have not managed to cure their incontinence. What has been missing is knowing the importance of this concept of bracing or engaging these muscles first prior to bending or coughing. It is also known as 'the knack' first described in 1998.[10]

My meaning of 'bracing' is:- prior to the increase in pressure pushing down on the bladder, internal organs and pelvic floor, you must first tighten your vagina and your anus to counteract this downward force. (If you feel lift in the vagina and anus with in-drawing of the low tummy then you can start by drawing your low tummy in first.)

Patients are often overwhelmed with the thought of having to do this with so many common activities. However, it is a habit or 'knack' which will become well-established and second nature with practise. Just as a young child is taught to cover their mouth with a cough or sneeze and, once it is learned, it becomes a very background action, *bracing* has to become a learned or trained response. It will also become much easier for you to remember as you feel improvement in your symptoms.

A word of caution:

Many women walk around all day *strongly tightening* their abdominal muscles having heard about the 'core' muscles or trying to have a flat tummy. This can lead to the pelvic floor muscles in some women becoming overly tight and can cause pelvic pain (known as *an overactive pelvic floor, a non-relaxing pelvic floor or levator myalgia, page 72*). So, firstly the action of the pelvic floor muscles is better if they are *gently* recruited and secondly be aware of *relaxing* your abdominal wall and pelvic floor muscles or *letting go* with them plenty of times through the day. Sometimes think of letting your muscles relax as though describing levels in an elevator and you want to *'relax to the ground floor and even to the basement'*.

If you have urinary leakage, prolapse or levator avulsion, brace or engage your muscles gently with all activities such as coughing, sneezing, laughing, lifting, jumping, squatting, bending over, pushing a heavy trolley etc. When there is a force from above, remember to give support from below. It's simply physics!

This is to remind you about using your muscles to counteract the downward forces of all those things that increase pressure in the abdomen. While pelvic floor muscle training is very important, learning how to pre-empt the increase in intra-abdominal pressure *(turning them on in time)* is what will prevent any stress urinary incontinence; will assist with minimising the risk of developing prolapse or worsening prolapse if they already have it; and will help prevent gas or bowel motion from escaping. Most importantly, this should assist with maintenance of any repair surgery.

A useful check to see if bracing is helping:
Sit on a firm wooden or plastic chair with your legs apart (Fig 7). First cough strongly **without bracing** and feel the descent of your pelvic floor into the chair. Then **brace strongly** and cough and feel how much more **stable** the pelvic floor feels.

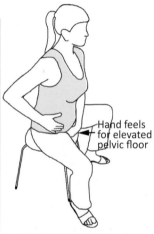

Hand feels for elevated pelvic floor

Fig 7. **Feel for descent when there is no bracing**
© Sue Croft 2018

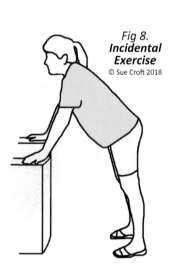

Fig 8.
Incidental Exercise
© Sue Croft 2018

Incidental Exercise:
Pelvic floor exercises can be done whilst waiting for the load of washing or dishwasher to finish (Fig 8). Stand leaning against the machine or a bench and gently draw in around the urethra/vagina - in this forward lean position you get better 'peri-urethral' sensation (around the urethra - the tube that brings the urine out).

Summary points

- *Do not hold your breath at all.* Learn to breathe normally as you do any exercise. This is very important. Learning to exhale on effort will protect your pelvic floor also rather than breath holding.

- *Do not try too hard at first and **stop if you sense any pushing down or bulging around the vagina**.* Check this by feeling with your hand. This is called bearing down and can make your prolapse or incontinence worse if you continue.

- *It's all about the **timing** and endurance of the muscles not just strength.* If you have had nerve damage or muscle avulsion (partial or complete rupturing of the muscle off the pubic bone see *page 16)* then we cannot cure that (at this point in time). So if your muscles are very weak, then it is imperative that you recruit *what is available* to you at the correct time.

- *Use reminders for your exercise session:* Perhaps use coloured stickers around the house to remind yourself, or when you clean your teeth, turn on the kettle or whenever you walk through a doorway. If you have poor sensation and difficulty in recruiting the muscles, then it is best to do your exercises in a quiet room, in a very focused way, so you are sure you are doing the exercises correctly. Using an image of the pelvic floor muscles will get your brain involved *(Fig 2, page 11)* and remember you do not have to get on the floor to exercise these muscles!

- *Remember to brace or engage before effort!* Gently draw in your pelvic floor muscles before and as you cough, sneeze, lift a weight (especially toddlers), get out of bed or a chair, particularly anything that is strenuous. It will become a life-long habit or 'knack'.

- *Relaxation* of your tummy and pelvic floor muscles is very important especially if you have any pelvic pain. Balance all tightening with plenty of relaxation.

- *Move so you decrease strains on your body.* When getting out of bed move through your side *(page 28, Fig 12);* divide heavy loads into smaller parcels; be aware when picking up toddlers (especially in the early days after a new baby); and teach young children to be independent to minimize lifting.

- *Regular pelvic floor muscle training is for life and can improve stress incontinence and severity of prolapse.* Incorporate these exercises into your activities of daily living.

- *Allow time for improvement* and ensure all strategies become life-time habits.

- *These strategies are for life!* So, to help you remember, do some diary or phone calendar entries every 3 months to prompt you to assess where you are at with your pelvic floor and think about having a review from a pelvic health physiotherapist yearly around the time of your birthday or other memorable dates. There are also many smart phone *apps* to help prompt you to do your pelvic floor exercises.

- *Get help from a:-*

  - *Pelvic health physiotherapist* if you are struggling with anything to do with your pelvic floor. Even though this is a very private area, so much difference can be made with proper help and careful and considered advice.

  - *Continence nurse or your general practice doctor* if living in rural areas where you may not be able to access a pelvic health physiotherapist.

  - *Specialist doctor* such as a urogynaecologist, gynaecologist, urologist and/or colorectal surgeon if these conservative measures are not successful at resolving your stress incontinence, prolapse or bowel issues. However, also be aware of the value of *'watchful waiting' (page 53)* and not rushing into surgery before all conservative strategies have been exhausted.

Hint: To help improve long-term compliance

If you sprain your ankle and see a physiotherapist for treatment, then when the ankle injury is healed, you never have to do those exercises again. However, with pelvic floor dysfunction, the treatment strategies taught by your physiotherapist are to be continued for life!

So to train this regularity, I tell my patients to make diary or calendar entries every 3 months for pelvic floor exercises to help remind them to do all the strategies in their program - bracing, pelvic floor muscle training, correct bladder & bowel positions, bladder retraining etc - forever. Anything to prompt you to keep a program going for the rest of your life.

The role of posture and the pelvic floor

Your posture influences your pelvic floor. When you hold erect posture, your pelvic floor activates; when you slump, your pelvic floor activity reduces. For many years, health professionals have directed that standing and sitting tall improves *'core stability'* and prevents joints like the sacro-iliac joints from *'going out'*. However, the importance of posture correction and holding a certain posture all the time has changed with more recent research. There is now evidence that *varying your posture* rather than always fixating on sitting tall and straight, is important to do. Sitting rigidly and constantly holding 'correct' posture can cause over-stiffening of the spinal and abdominal muscles and importantly can *generate a fear that not holding a certain posture will lead to increased back and pelvic pain.* In fact the reverse is true.[24]

Nevertheless, there is a relationship between posture and the pelvic floor, which you can use in different circumstances to your advantage.

- For this awareness check, it is best to sit on a firm chair or stool either wooden or plastic with your legs apart and your back away from the back of the chair *(Fig 9)*. This is to increase your awareness of the relationship between your tummy and pelvic floor. When you sit tall, your low tummy and pelvic floor muscles naturally and gently engage and may assist to hold any prolapse up and in and increase urethral closing pressure.[25] In this posture practise maintaining relaxed breathing and perform *'the knack'* as you cough, feeling the support the pelvic floor provides you.

- When slumped in a chair, now feel the relaxation of the belly and you may feel relaxation of the pelvic floor into the chair.

- If you have any persistent pelvic pain, it is important to regularly practice relaxing your tummy and pelvic floor to 'down-train' these muscles and decrease any tightness they may have. Let your tummy go without slumping and do some tummy breaths feeling the tummy rise under your hand as you breathe in and fall away as you breathe out. This *belly breathing* is also a helpful strategy to reduce anxiety.

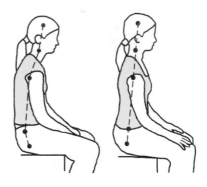

Fig 9. It's ok to vary your posture
© Sue Croft 2018

As women age, particularly if they have osteoporosis, they can become more rounded through their back and shoulders and lose height. Doing a morning stretch can help to help maintain good flexibility and length of muscles and prevent a thoracic kyphosis (often called a Dowager's hump). *Fight gravity!*

Stand against a wall or closed door *(Fig 10).* Look at a point on the opposite wall in line with your eyes straight ahead (not up or down) Feet are back against the wall, buttocks touching, shoulders touching and the back of your head touching without losing that spot on the wall in front. (If your neck and upper back are stiff and you can't reach the wall with your head, don't tilt your head backwards to touch the wall.)

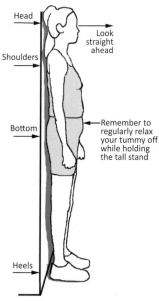

Do this regularly, not only as a postural stretch but as an indicator that you might be starting to get stiffness and tightness in your muscles. *Do not* force your neck back if you have pain or any nerve pressure signs such as pins and needles or numbness. If you do have pins and needles or numbness, then you should check with your physiotherapist before you attempt this postural check. Hold the position for around 10 to 20 secs and then roll your shoulders and neck forward and relax them.

Fig 10. **Wall standing posture stretch**
© Sue Croft 2018

A **cobra stretch** *(Fig 11)* is also a good stretch for the cervical and thoracic spine if you can lie down on your tummy. Start by just lying on your tummy and place your hands up at shoulder height and then push up gently– if you are stiff gradually go a little further each day. Evidence also tells us that strengthening your back extensor muscles (lifting your head and shoulders up with your arms beside your body) is good for osteoporosis prevention, provides a significant reduction in vertebral fractures and helps balance and falls reduction.[26]

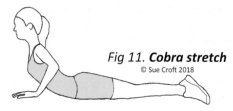

Fig 11. **Cobra stretch**
© Sue Croft 2018

26

Lifting with pelvic floor dysfunction

We need to lift objects in our activities of daily living. We need to lift children, bags of potting mix and groceries amongst other things. Lifting weights helps maintain bone density. Minimising forces generated by increased intra-abdominal pressure (IAP) with lifting is important to prevent recurrence of prolapse and protect any repair surgery. The evidence in the research is variable about the pressures generated with lifting but some key points to consider:

- *Understand about the state of your pelvic floor:* Do you have levator avulsion? Are your PF muscles weak? Do you have a collagen issue? (See *page 48*) These factors will influence your decision about what weight you can lift up to.
- *If you have significant levator avulsion* (poor pelvic floor support, *page 16*) *and an enlarged distance between your urethra and anus* (normal is less than 7cm - this measurement is called GH+PB Valsalva, *page 17)*, then you have a greater risk of developing prolapse and potentially further increasing your risk of worsening your prolapse with lifting heavy. This measurement can be assessed and explained by your pelvic health physiotherapist. Learn to pre-contract your pelvic floor prior to lifting (*'the knack'* or bracing) and a supporting pessary may splint and protect when lifting (discuss with your doctor).
- Minimize heavy lifting in the first 3 months post surgical repair.
- Pressures are highest when lifting from a squat position. In one study lifting 0kg (nothing) with a squat manoeuvre generated more intra-abdominal pressure than lifting 10kg off the counter or receiving 15kg into outstretched hands. Based on this, having children handed to you rather than squatting to the ground to lift them (post-op) may generate less IAP (called the receive manoeuvre).[27]
- Intra-abdominal pressures generated were significantly greater in obese women than those who were not obese, so there may be a need for greater care with lifting if you are overweight.[28]
- Do not hold your breath - *keep breathing while lifting*.
- If you have had any repair surgery, there is no evidence in the literature definitively supporting any specific weight avoidance with lifting, at this point in time. The consensus amongst urogynaecologists varies from 5 kg to 15kg maximum weight for lifting from 12 weeks on post-surgery. It is important to check with your own surgeon. If you are lifting young children after your surgery or have a job which requires higher impact activities, there may be a place for discussing the use of a pessary post-operatively with your surgeon, as a further preventative strategy (after your stitches have completely dissolved, when no pain and with close consultation with your surgeon).
- Lifting weights helps with bone density - discuss the pros and cons with your pelvic health physiotherapist.

With prolapse, following repair surgery or when there's abdominal separation

One of the most repetitive things we do over a lifetime is to get in and out of bed and if you have stress urinary incontinence, prolapse, repair surgery or an abdominal muscle separation post-natally, manoeuvring as described below can save significant downward forces on the pelvic floor and prevent worsening abdominal separation.

- Firstly, while lying on your back, tighten your pelvic floor muscles and draw your knees up one at a time. Make sure you have enough room between your body and the edge of the bed to roll without falling out. Maintain the pelvic floor contraction and roll onto your side keeping your shoulders, hips and bent legs in line *(Fig 12)*.

- If you have rolled to the left side for example, dig your left elbow into the bed and push through your right hand, gently lowering your legs over the edge of the bed. Do the opposite for rolling to the right side.

- This method of getting in and out of bed is also useful if you have a rectus diastasis (abdominal muscle separation while pregnant or after childbirth) or have any type of hernia.

- To lie down from sitting, basically do the opposite of getting out of bed. It helps if you put both hands to the same side, and then lie down onto that side, then contract your pelvic floor and roll onto your back.

- This method of getting in and out of bed is what you will use in hospital after you have had your repair surgery.

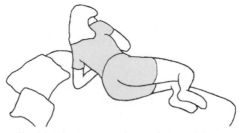

Fig 12. How to get in and out of bed
© Sue Croft 2018

Chapter 3

Causes of pelvic health issues

There are a myriad of pelvic health conditions, such as, incontinence, prolapse, bowel dysfunction and pelvic pain. Some risk factors are listed below but there are many others which can cause problems.

You may be at risk of having problems with your pelvic health if you have:

- *Had bladder or bowel problems as a child.*
- *Had endometriosis or painful periods.*
- *Been pregnant.*
- *Delivered vaginally.*
- *Had a caesarean section.*
- *Had gynaecological surgery.*
- *Had bowel issues: chronic constipation, long-term straining to pass a bowel motion or chronic diarrhoea.*
- *Gained excess weight.*
- *Worked out hard at the gym especially doing heavy weight training.*
- *Played a lot of high impact sports over your lifetime.*
- *Done lots of sit-ups as part of a boot camp or training program.*
- *Done repeated double leg lifts in an exercise program.*
- *Have chronic low back pain, sacro-iliac joint (SIJ) or hip pain.*
- *Reached menopause .*
- *Had a chronic cough.*
- *Suffered with hay fever, sneezing regularly and violently.*
- *Needed prolonged bed rest.*
- *Had gynaecological cancer*
- *Undergone chemotherapy for any type of cancer*
- *A low level of exercise.*
- *A very sedentary job.*
- *Worked in strenuous jobs (which involve lifting heavy weights).*
- *Reached your seventies, eighties or nineties - ageing!*

Signs of a weakened pelvic floor and /or bladder dysfunction?

- Any leakage of urine with increased intra-abdominal pressure (IAP) - extra pressure from coughing, sneezing, bending, laughing, lifting weights, exercise - *see box below*. A hard cough can generate a transient increase of IAP of 150cmH$_2$O or more which is very significant.
- Any leakage of urine when hurrying to the toilet, on hearing running water or putting a key in the door when arriving home.
- Leakage of urine after standing up off the toilet after voiding.
- Insidious leakage not fitting into the previous categories.
- Increased frequency of urination (normal should be approximately 5 to 7 times during the day and once at night for drinking 2 litres of fluid – you will need to go more times if you have a higher fluid intake. (See *page 35* for good bladder habits)
- Dragging or aching sensation around the vagina or anus which can be due to prolapse (relaxation) of the pelvic organs. See *Chapter 5* - What is Prolapse? Pelvic pain can also be due to overly tight pelvic floor muscles.
- Problems in controlling wind or bowel contents (anal flatus or faecal incontinence).
- Chronic constipation due to difficulty in emptying your bowels causing a need to strain. (This is also known as obstructed defaecation – see bowel management section, *Chapter 6).*
- Decreased sexual awareness or sensation.

What causes increases in intra-abdominal pressure?
- *Going from sit to stand*
- *Bending over*
- *Coughing, sneezing*
- *Lifting and squatting*
- *Pushing (trolleys, prams)*
- *Jumping (on the trampoline; at aerobics)*
- *Jogging*
- *Blowing your nose*
- *Vomiting*
- *Straining with bowels*
- *Bearing down with orgasm*
- *Laughing strongly*
- *Blowing up balloons*
- *Sit ups and double leg lifts*

Chapter 4

Normal and abnormal bladder function

Normal Bladder Function

The adult bladder (under 70 years of age), should store 350 to 500 mls filling passively - that is, the bladder should not spasm and contract during filling. At 350 to 500 mls, it should provide a stretch message to your brain telling you your bladder is full. When you are ready to void, it should then empty completely to a nil or low residual.

There should be no urgency, no urge leakage (incontinence), no pain, no need to strain to empty and the flow should be continuous and steady, with a flow rate of around 20 to 30 mls per second and no dribble or leak afterwards. See *Chapter 16,* for the effects on urinary function with ageing.

Common bladder problems

These definitions are from the International Continence Society [29] :-

- *Stress Incontinence (SUI)* - is a complaint of involuntary loss of urine on effort or physical exertion *(see page 30).*

- *Overactive Bladder (OAB)* - is an urgency, with or without urge incontinence, usually with frequency and nocturia (see below).

- *Urge Incontinence* - is an involuntary leakage of urine with an urgent urge to go to the toilet often associated with triggers such as key in the door, running water, seeing the toilet, filling the kettle, high anxiety situations etc.

- *Bladder Urgency* - is a complaint of a sudden compelling desire to pass urine which is difficult to defer.

- *Urinary Frequency* - is when you are voiding more than 5 to 7 times from when you get up in the morning to when you go to bed at night when drinking 2 litres of fluid total in a day.

- *Nocturia* - is a complaint of interruption of sleep one or more times because of the need to micturate (pass urine). Each void is preceded and followed by sleep.

31

- *Unconscious insensible leakage* - is the complaint of involuntary loss of urine unaccompanied by either urgency or stress incontinence provocative factors. The only awareness of the incontinence episode is the feeling of wetness due to the urine. It is also known as *insidious leakage* - and can be due to poor urethral closing pressure when post-menopausal (a deficient urethral sphincter) and can be assisted by using local oestrogen in the vagina twice a week (can also present when breast feeding). Check with your doctor to see if local oestrogen may be helpful for you and not contra-indicated.

- *Post-micturition dribble* - means the loss of a few drops of urine after the main stream when the bladder appears to be empty. It occurs in women, but it is also common in men.

- *Nocturnal enuresis* is the complaint of loss of urine occurring during sleep (wetting the bed).

- *Voiding Dysfunction* - is when the bladder doesn't empty properly and the resulting residuals can cause urinary tract infections and/or urinary frequency. The flow can be hesitant or staccato (start-stop-start).

- *Recurrent Urinary Tract Infections* - This diagnosis is by clinical history assisted by the results of diagnostic tests involving the determination of the occurrence of more than one symptomatic and medically diagnosed urinary tract infection (UTI) over the previous 12 months. It can often be caused by incomplete emptying of the bladder; can be related to sexual intercourse; can sometimes follow gynaecological surgery; is common in post-menopausal women with an atrophic vagina (decreased oestrogen causing fragile tissue quality and poorer tone and a rigid 'drainpipe' urethra which allows bacteria to enter the bladder); or is seen in patients who suffer regular episodes of faecal soiling. Local oestrogen pessaries or creams can often help with this condition. Discuss with your doctor.

- *Bladder Pain Syndrome (BPS)* - used to be known as Interstitial Cystitis - is defined as chronic (>6 months) pelvic pain, pressure or discomfort perceived to be related to the urinary bladder accompanied by at least one other urinary symptom such as persistent urge to void or frequency in the absence of proven obvious pathology (urinary tract infections). Distinctive signs on cystoscopy (a camera that is inserted in the bladder) such as pinpoint-sized areas of bleeding (glomerulations) and Hunner's ulcers in the bladder wall may be seen.

Some useful bladder hints

- Always use the correct position to urinate (page 34).

- Always take your time to urinate, never strain, just completely relax your tummy and pelvic floor.

- When finished urinating, wipe from front to back.

- Wear cotton underwear or ones with a full cotton gusset in them to help prevent vaginal/perineal irritation from synthetic materials.

- Wash your underwear with a sensitive laundry liquid.

- If you need a bath for relaxation, shower first, then bathe and avoid using bubble baths and bath 'bombs'.

- If you are prone to recurrent urinary tract infections (UTI's) perhaps reduce or avoid having frequent baths because of risk of irritation of the urethra and UTIs.

- If prone to recurrent UTIs that are related to sexual intercourse then remember to urinate before and after intercourse and always use a lubricant to reduce drying of the vagina and reduce friction with prolonged penetration.

- There is evidence that a preventative dose (1 to 2 tablets only) of an antibiotic taken after intercourse may prevent UTI's.[30] Speak with your doctor.

- There is evidence that drinking 1.5 litres of water after sex decreased the risk of UTIs in those women prone to recurrent UTIs, but of course this is a significant amount of water (or other fluid) to drink at one time. If you are plagued by recurrent UTIs you may like to try it.[31]

- If post-menopausal, local oestrogen pessaries or cream can help urogenital function particularly UTIs. Speak with your doctor.

- Cranberry tablets have been shown to be nearly as effective as long-term low dose antibiotics for UTI prevention in women (and do not contribute to antibiotic resistance).[32]

- Have breaks if using cranberry to prevent UTIs, as long-term use can be linked with increased production of kidney stones.[33]

Position for emptying your bladder

- This position shown in the images below enhances the emptying of your bladder and should be used for life.
- Keep the natural curve in your back, with your chest out of waistline - not slumped.
- Lean forward at the hips, lean on your hands which are placed on your knees.
- Sit with your knees wide apart, feet flat on the floor.
- **Relax your tummy and pelvic floor muscles** and look straight ahead when about to start passing urine.
- Take your time, ensure you are emptying without straining.
- When the flow is finished, wipe front to back, gently draw in your tummy and pelvic floor as you stand and walk away.
- If you have a confirmed history of a voiding dysfunction (not emptying your bladder properly) then you may be advised by your health professional to do a *'double void'* (to stand and then sit and void again).
- Young children who sit to void should have foot support until their legs are long enough to reach the floor with hips and knees both at 90 degrees to help ensure their bladder is emptying fully.

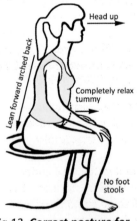

Fig 13. **Correct posture for emptying bladder**

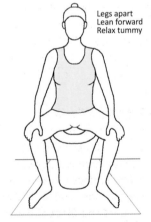

Fig 14. **Correct posture for emptying bladder**

Important:

This position is particularly important post-operatively if there is a slow or start-stop-start flow of urine due to swelling. Resist the temptation to strain to urinate as this may contribute to failure of your surgery.

34

Good bladder habits for life

Simple changes to your lifetime habits such as following these good bladder habits can make significant improvements to your urinary control. Sometimes our family members have been responsible for passing down rituals and beliefs about bladder and bowel health which are not accurate and lead us into bad habits with our urinary and bowel function. Surprisingly, it is not as hard as it may seem to make these changes.

- *Drink approximately 2 litres of fluid per day as a general rule* (which can include water, juice, milk and decaffeinated tea/coffee) - and more if exercising or breastfeeding. The actual amount required in a average temperature day with no physical activity can be calculated by the equation 24 mls per kilogram of bodyweight. Avoid fluids with artificial sugar such as nutra-sweet, as this can irritate the bladder. Water is always best rather than highly sugared drinks, especially in view of their calorie content. Avoid drinking too much fluid (overdrinking can be a problem).

- *For that 2 litres* you should go to the toilet *5 to 7 times* to pass urine (from when you get up out of bed in the morning to when you go to bed at night) and *0 to 1 at night.* You will need to go more often if you drink more fluid.

- *Caffeine is an irritant of the bladder. Restrict caffeine* to 3 cups per day if you have no urgency, urge incontinence or faecal incontinence symptoms. Try to *eliminate caffeine* if you have urinary or faecal urgency, frequency or control problems. Decrease your caffeine intake *slowly* to avoid a withdrawal headache. There are many brands of decaffeinated tea and coffee.

- *Some Australian brands which have a decaffeinated alternative:*
  - Teas - Twinings, Tetley, Lipton, Dilmah, Rooibos, Yorkshire decaf teabags. Most herbal teas have no caffeine (anecdotally, peppermint tea may increase urgency).
  - Instant coffees - Nescafe, Moccona instant decafeinated coffee.
  - Plunger and coffee machine coffee - Vittoria, Lavazza, Fair Trade, Grinders and Black Sheep are chemical free (at the time of writing). Pod machines always have a decaffeinated pod available.
  - For other countries, check for your local decaffeinated brands.

- *Remember alcohol is a diuretic, a bladder irritant and muscle relaxant* and is likely to make urgency, frequency and urge urinary incontinence problems worse.

- *Cut out the 'just in case' visits to the toilet.* Go to the toilet when you have a *full bladder sensation* (above the pubic hair region), rather than the first urethral sensation (around the urethra). Do your measures with your bladder diary to become more familiar with 350 to 500 mls capacities, the normal adult capacity. Always use your common sense with this so as not to have unfortunate accidents if caught in a traffic jam!

- *You can over-fill your bladder.* Teachers, hairdressers and nurses are just some of the professions who notoriously over-hold with their bladders. The daytime maximum capacity of your bladder should be 500 mls. Many women wake with a very full bladder - this is unavoidable, but try and avoid overholding while you are awake during the day.

- *Use the correct position for passing urine (Figs 13 and 14).* Never 'hover' or 'perch' to urinate as you may not empty your bladder properly. Use a *purse pack of antiseptic wipes* to clean the seat down prior to urinating if you are anxious about sitting on a public toilet seat.

- However, if you feel your flow rate is slower with this position use the position which feels better and has the lowest residual. This can be checked with a post-void ultrasound.

- *Never strain to empty.* Relax your tummy and pelvic floor and let the bladder do the emptying.

- A significant vaginal prolapse can cause your urine flow to be slow. Sometimes being fitted with a pessary to reduce your prolapse can significantly help your flow rate and bladder emptying.

- *All your life have good bowel function.* Refer to *Chapter 6*.

Don't forget!

*Caffeine can irritate the smooth muscle of the bowel as well as the bladder and be a cause of **bowel urgency** and **soiling**. If this is the case experiment with decaffeinated teas and coffee and see if this helps reduce your faecal incontinence. However, for some people with chronic constipation and no bladder urgency symptoms, caffeine can be useful to help stimulate the bowels if they are sluggish in the morning.*

Caffeine levels in fluids and foods

Coke Classic
36mg
per 375ml

Diet Coke
48mg
per 375ml

Red Bull
80mg
per 250ml

Mother Energy Drink
160mg
per 500ml

Dark Chocolate
30mg
per 50g

Hot chocolate
5-10mg
per 250ml

1 cup
instant coffee
60-80mg
per 250ml

1 shot
espresso coffee
(cafe quality)
194mg

1 cup
black tea
48mg
250ml

Caffeine levels in common fluids and foods

Source: Journal of Food Science 2010; 75(3):R77-87,
Australian Institute of Sport
© Sue Croft 2018

Common bladder tests that might be performed

There are a number of tests that may be undertaken if you have any of these bladder conditions. These tests will help ascertain which bladder problems you have and help formulate appropriate treatment.

Bladder Diary
A bladder diary is a simple and a very effective test that gives the doctor, the physiotherapist, continence nurse and the patient considerable information about bladder function. It can tell you your bladder capacity, frequency of urination, episodes of leakage, degree of urgency, daily fluid intake, times when drinking occurs, volume and type of fluid intake. Complete a 48 hour diary for your treating health professional and also for your own benefit - you can learn so much from completing a bladder diary. See *Appendix 2* for an example and *Appendix 3* for a blank form. Remember over-holding your bladder volumes (not the first one of the day) can be a problem if greater than 500 mls.

Renal Ultrasound
An ultrasound assesses kidney function and can be used to check pre and post bladder volumes to see if the bladder empties completely on urinating.

Micro-urine
A simple test to check if there is an infection in the urine. If symptoms of urgency and frequency change suddenly when there is no pain or feeling of being unwell, it is always important to check for infection - particularly after any repair surgery when the bladder may not be emptying completely.

Urodynamics
A test that uses a small catheter inserted into the bladder to fill it with fluid to study the function of the bladder and urethra during filling and urinating. It reports about the function of the smooth muscle of the bladder called the detrusor muscle, which is responsible for emptying the bladder and about urethral sphincter function.

Alert!
*If you get a **sudden change** in your urinary control such as frequency, urgency or urge leakage, then always think urinary tract infection (UTI) and go to your doctor and get a micro-urine test performed. You do not always have a temperature, pass blood or have pain with urinating to have a UTI!*

Treatment strategies for stress incontinence (SUI)

While the urethral sphincter is the primary mechanism for preventing incontinence during increased intra-abdominal pressure, it is helped by the pelvic floor muscles. The urethral sphincter is made up of striated (voluntary) and smooth muscle fibres.[11] Any changes in the ability of the smooth muscle sphincter mechanisms to provide good urethral closing pressure will contribute significantly to stress incontinence and insidious leakage. The urethral sphincter mechanism also deteriorates with ageing due to decreased vascularity and will benefit from oestrogen supplements locally to help with maintaining closing pressure after menopause. Discuss with your doctor.

The treatment strategies for stress urinary incontinence involve:-

- *Extensive education* about normal and abnormal pelvic health

- *Pelvic floor muscle training (PFMT)* as described on *page 10.*

- *'The knack' or bracing* is important with all increases in intra-abdominal pressure such as coughing, sneezing, laughing, lifting, blowing your nose, on initially pushing your shopping trolley when loaded, squatting, jumping, gardening, rowing, repetitive bending and so the list goes on. Anytime there is pressure pushing down you should learn 'the knack' or habit of contracting the support mechanism from below - *the pelvic floor muscles.*

- *Internal Splints*
    - For more vigorous activities such as walking briskly, jogging and sport, women have found that using a tampon as a splint for the activity may keep you dry and may also assist with holding up any prolapse **(read the guidelines on the tampon packaging particularly with reference to Toxic Shock Syndrome TSS, before deciding to use a tampon in this way).** Think carefully about this option and make your own considered decision. Always remove the tampon after the activity. If you are post-menopausal you may find the tampon drying and it may help to use lubricant on the tip of the tampon or speak to your doctor about commencing local oestrogen cream. Check with your doctor before using a tampon as an internal splint if you have any concerns.
    - A device called a *'Contiform'®* is a type of pessary specifically for treatment of stress urinary incontinence. They are manufactured from medical-grade elastomeric material, that is removed every night. The manufacturer recommends that it should not be used in conjunction with a Mirena® (a type of contraceptive device). While they are often very successful at treating stress incontinence, each one has a limited

lifespan as they break in the front rim after a certain number of uses and need to be replaced. They come in 3 sizes - small, medium and large. You cannot use either a tampon or Contiform® for 3 months after any repair surgery. Your pelvic health physiotherapist may be able to supply and fit the Contiform®.

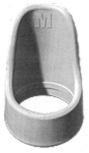

Contiform®

♦ There are other types of continence pessaries available that can help with stress urinary incontinence. They are called a *continence dish* and a *ring with knob*. These can be fitted by a urogynaecologist, gynaecologist, some general practitioners and many pelvic health physiotherapists. The protrusion at the front of the pessary gives compression to the urethra to stop urinary leakage with effort. The continence pessaries with a platform often stay in place better.

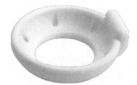

Continence dish
(no platform)

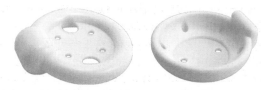

Continence pessaries with platforms

Treatment strategies for the overactive bladder (OAB) (including frequency, urgency and urge incontinence)

The role of the bladder is to store to around 350 to 500 mls of urine. However, sometimes through: bad habits, stress and anxiety, drinking too much caffeine or alcohol, and gynaecological surgery, the ability of the bladder to store urine passively may deteriorate and the bladder wall starts to spasm as it fills. This is called an overactive bladder and gives the patient the symptoms of *urgency, frequency,* with or without *urge leakage.*

The treatment strategy for these symptoms is called *bladder retraining (also known as bladder drill, bladder training, bladder re-education).*[34]

Bladder retraining is the technique used to:

* try to increase the capacity of the bladder and to store urine to the normal adult capacity of 350 to 500 mls. Holding larger volumes than the maximum of 500 mls should be avoided where possible (except perhaps for the first void of the day). Certain professions such as teachers, hairdressers and nurses often over-hold more than 500 mls because they can never leave their classroom, shop or ward to get to a toilet. Repeatedly holding large capacities beyond 500 mls can lead to other bladder dysfunction.

* decrease the sensitivity of the bladder.

* retrain your bladder to store urine without giving you urgent, uncomfortable spasms in your bladder or urge leakage.

* give you more time between voids (wees), more freedom to go out without constantly seeking the nearest toilet and constantly changing pads and most importantly, less anxiety and more confidence with your bladder function.

The process of bladder retraining :

* *Find out what your bladder capacity is.* Refer to *Appendix 2* for an example of how to fill in a *Bladder Diary* and then copy the blank form in *Appendix 3* and follow the directions to fill it in over 48 hours. This will tell you how much work you have to do with your bladder.

* *Know if you empty your bladder completely* before undertaking bladder deferral. This can be checked by a pre and post void (wee) ultrasound by a pelvic health physiotherapist or a radiology centre.

* *Then if you are trying to increase the capacity of your bladder to the normal volume of 350 to 500 mls,* when you get the first urge to go, try and defer, hold on longer to increase the capacity of the bladder (as long as it is not **too** long already since you last went). Refer to the good bladder habits on *page 35.*

41

- *Use the urge control techniques (see below) to help you defer.* These are techniques which are like 'tricks' which work in four ways to help you with the symptoms that come under the umbrella of an overactive bladder. It is no use asking your brain to defer the urge without having some strategies to help you control this strong desire to go.

Urge control techniques

The four ways the urge control techniques work:
- By turning off the urge through a reflex.
- Via inhibition of the sacral nerve pathways.
- Through muscle control (engaging the pelvic floor muscles).
- Via distraction of the brain and diverting your attention from the bladder.

These are the urge control techniques (tricks) to help you turn off the urge:
- *Using perineal or clitoral pressure such as:*
  - *Hand pressure over the perineum (the area around the vagina), clitoris and/or urethra (suitable for when you are by yourself).*
  - *Sitting on the edge of a chair or table.*
  - *Sitting on a rolled up towel when in the car (on a long car trip).*
  - *Sitting on the edge of the bed prior to getting out of bed first thing in the morning.*
- *Crossing your thighs in standing or sitting (achieves the same as perineal or clitoral pressure if out in public).*
- *Buttock tightening and toe curling. These strategies work by using the sacral nerve pathways to over-ride the sensory messages to the bladder - not because you are holding on with those muscles.*
- *A gentle pelvic floor muscle hold or gentle tummy draw-in. This works by direct muscle activation of the urethral sphincter and pelvic floor muscles.*

Do one (or all of these strategies) to help calm the desire to urinate. Once the initial urge has passed, then if your bladder is **not** very full because you have been to the toilet recently, just get on with doing your tasks and activities such as folding, filing, computer work or ironing - that is, *get on with life.*

When the next (second) urge comes, if you feel it is *still* too soon and you want to defer again, do the same thing - use the urge control techniques to defer the urge which will further help you to build up your bladder capacity.

This continues until either you feel it is time to go because your bladder is full or you are too stressed to continue deferring. It is definitely important to progress slowly so you don't feel like you are failing by having wetting incidents. Take your time to improve your bladder capacity.

If you have successfully held on for a number of hours and *have a full bladder*, you may suffer urge leakage (wet yourself) if you try and go to the toilet with that strong urge. So to avoid urge leakage - *stop, breathe and don't panic* and *use the urge control tricks on the previous page,* to yet again turn off the urge to urinate. Once the urge has settled then use the following strategies to *get to the toilet dry*. In the early days of your bladder retraining, it may help you to feel less anxious about deferring if you wear a pad. As your confidence builds and your capacities get bigger, then you can discard the pad.

How to get to the toilet dry when you have a full bladder:

- *Stand carefully* (if you have been sitting), keep your chest loose and gently pull in your pelvic floor.
- *Breathe easily* and walk quietly to the toilet - *do not hold your breath*.
- *Counting the steps* may help to divert attention and use any other *distraction techniques* you can.
- *It takes time to retrain your bladder* when you have been going with small capacities for a long time. So be *patient, consistent and persistent* with these strategies. Don't give up if you have some accidents. Look at the big picture. Having a major accident is very distressing and often that is your focus, but what you must ask yourself is - are you generally getting better as the weeks go on?

Timed voiding

How to bladder retrain if the sensation of urgency is debilitating and not responding to the above bladder training: Timed voiding

If you are suffering with *significant sensory urgency* or finding that holding on is making you *anxious* or *giving you bladder pain*, then undertake a program of *timed voiding* to manage this. Firstly, complete a bladder diary and note the time frame between voids (wees) and aim to go to the toilet a short time before the urges are arriving. If the strong urge arrives at 2 hours then go to the toilet *without an urge to go* at 1 hour 50 minutes to avoid the unpleasant, anxiety-inducing sensation of an urgent urge. As you come to find this easier, you can increase the length of time between voids.

This will allow you to decrease the unpleasant sensory urgency you are experiencing. *Prompted timed voiding* is also useful if you are caring for someone with cognitive issues such as dementia.

Medications:

There are a number of medications to assist with the overactive bladder by decreasing the severity of the urge and the amount of urge leakage and to help with nocturia. They are often very helpful in retraining the bladder. I liken them to using training wheels when learning to ride a bike. Once your bladder has retrained, then you can often wean off the medication.

These medications are prescribed by your specialist or general practitioner. Older medications have side effects such as a dry mouth and have to be used with care with narrow-angle glaucoma but newer generation medications have less debilitating side effects. Some anticholinergics should be prescribed with care to the older age group because of their side effects with dementia.

Some medications (both oral and patches) are available on the national government subsidy schemes and make them more affordable. Check with your doctor or specialist to see if these will be helpful. If you see a specialist, urodynamic testing of the bladder will demonstrate if these drugs might help your problem.

Nocturia

Nocturia (when you are getting up to urinate once or more at night after you have initially gone to sleep) can be very debilitating and often worsens with ageing. Apart from your sleep being affected, in the frail elderly there can be an increased risk of falls on attempting to go to the toilet at night. Multiple medical conditions are associated with nocturia and therefore thorough investigation is critical to find out the cause of nocturia.[35] The first test to do is a 2 day bladder diary which must include all night-time voids to assess your night-time total voided volume and compare it to your daytime total voids.

This will show if there is polyuria which is excessive urine production. *Nocturnal polyuria* is defined as nocturnal urine production greater than 33% of your total 24hr urine output, at any age.[36] You can calculate this out by totalling your night time output and divide it into the total urine production for the whole day.

The diary could also reveal that your bladder has a reduced capacity to store urine during sleep compared to during the day. Testing for both types of diabetes and doing a formal sleep study to assess for sleep apnoea are also useful investigations.

Treatment strategies for managing nocturia:

- Have a thorough medical review to eliminate treatable medical conditions such as heart disease, peripheral artery disease, diabetes, sleep apnoea and others which can also contribute to nocturia.
- Reduce your fluid intake around dinner time.
- Wear compression calf stockings during the day to assist with reducing leg swelling and improve daytime output.
- Have a daytime lie down, with your compression calf socks on and pump your ankles up and down. Void once you get up and walk around.
- Discuss scheduling your heart medications (such as diuretics) for earlier in the day with your doctor .
- Have a sleep study if you have signs of sleep apnoea (snoring, periodic limb movements, waking feeling exhausted, feeling like you could fall asleep when driving).
- There is a new medication for adult nocturnal polyuria which you could discuss with your doctor.

Alert:

When you complete your bladder dairy, it may show that you are only voiding small urine volumes. However sometimes this can be actually due to not emptying your bladder completely. Therefore if you try to build up the voided volumes by deferring, you will potentially be holding too much urine in your bladder (more than 500 mls). To assess if you are not emptying your bladder completely, a **pre and post void ultrasound** *checks your residual urine and is a non-invasive and useful test to have performed. Your physiotherapist may perform this or ask your doctor for a referral to a radiology facility to have this test and perhaps a referral to a specialist to assess the severity of the bladder problem.*

Summary points

- Normal bladder capacity is between 350 to 500 mls. Know yours by doing a 48 hour bladder diary. Repeat every couple of years to pick up any deterioration in the storage capacity of your bladder.

- A pre-void and post-void ultrasound of your bladder will alert you to any residual urine left after voiding.

- Good bladder habits are lifelong habits. Remember the concept of deferment and avoid doing small, *'just in case'* voids forever.

- Drink around 2 litres of fluid per day including water, decaffeinated drinks, juice and milk, more if it is hot or you are exercising or breast feeding. The minimum amount of fluid you need to drink can be roughly calculated at 24 mls/kilo of weight for 24 hours. Be aware that *over-drinking* can cause problems.

- Your bladder capacity can decrease as you age. Frequency particularly nocturia (frequency at night) can be very annoying and debilitating in the elderly as they suffer very interrupted sleep and this leads to daytime exhaustion.

- Eliminate bladder irritants such as caffeine, nutra-sweet and alcohol if you have urgency, frequency, urge leakage or nocturia. Test for a month without these irritants and assess if you have improved. Then *you* decide whether to continue with restriction or elimination of these products depending on your results.

- Teach all children and grandchildren the correct information. Many women with poor bladder capacities inadvertently teach their children the wrong bladder behaviours based on their own experiences. It is important for children to go to the toilet on the 'bouncy full bladder' message - not go at your convenience or 'just in case' and always have foot support for young children sitting on the toilet whenever possible.

Chapter **5**

What is prolapse?

Vaginal prolapse occurs when there is a relaxation of the fascia and other ligamentous supports of the vagina causing the organs of the pelvis (the bladder, uterus and bowel) to descend. The prolapse can be mild, moderate or extend beyond the introitus (the opening of the vagina). It is strongly associated with levator avulsion *(page 16)*. There can also be rectal prolapse when the lining of the rectum protrudes out of the anus. Vaginal and rectal prolapse may require surgery if conservative physiotherapy strategies have not controlled the symptoms a woman is suffering.

Women commonly complain about :
- the feeling of a lump or bulge in the vagina or dropping below the entrance to the vagina (feeling like a dislodged tampon). There may be rubbing of the tissue against the underwear causing ulceration.
- a sense of vaginal drag, heaviness or ache.
- low back pain.
- a change with sexual intercourse (a change in the 'look' of the vagina causing anxiety for the woman, a bulky feeling; even difficulty achieving penetration, or a loose, lax feeling during intercourse).
- the inability to hold a tampon in.
- a loose feeling when exercising.
- difficulty with complete evacuation of the bowels.
- some rectal tissue coming out of the rectum during or after defaecation.
- difficulty getting clean after defaecation.

Women are often devastated on learning that they have a prolapse. It is a very common condition with up to 50% of women who have had a vaginal delivery suffering from vaginal prolapse throughout their lifetime.[5] However, many prolapses are asymptomatic for many years. It is important that women know if they have levator avulsion so they can implement the strategies in this book to prevent a prolapse from occurring or worsening of any diagnosed prolapse.

This need not be considered a devastating diagnosis. You have read many preventative strategies already and there are many more to come in this book - this knowledge is empowering. It is important not to catastrophise about your prolapse as this will change your life if you become fearful about moving and exercising. Decreasing your exercise can also affect your mood making you feel depressed and have a significant impact on your quality of life and that of your family. Seek help early and find yourself a prolapse mentor - a health professional who will give you evidence-based advice and treatment as well as supporting you emotionally should you need it.

With increasing awareness about prolapse, many women are worried they have prolapse, when in fact they don't. This causes tremendous anxiety, perhaps completely unnecessarily. It is important to get a diagnosis confirmed by your doctor or pelvic health physiotherapist.

Sometimes prolapse does progress, is very significant and requires further intervention. Approximately 10% of women require surgery at some stage in their life.[5] Up to 30% of the women who have had surgery will require re-operation.[5] If the woman has had a muscle tear (levator avulsion) at the time of her vaginal delivery the failure rate for surgery can be up to 80% [37] which of course is a very disturbing statistic and makes the information about preventative strategies even more important. Levator avulsion is extensively described on *page 16*. While vaginal and rectal prolapse is definitely associated with having a vaginal delivery, it can be seen in nulliparous women (no children) as it is strongly associated with a history of straining with your bowels.

Collagen type is also important in the link with prolapse and incontinence. If you have the poorer type of collagen, then you can be predisposed to suffering with prolapse and other pelvic floor dysfunction.[38] You or your daughters[39] may have excelled at gymnastics at school but this *hyper-mobility* or *hyper-flexibility* can be an indicator to your future predisposition to prolapse and could also cause problems such as:

- early low back pain in pregnancy.
- marked abdominal striae in pregnancy (stretch marks).
- developing a significant rectus diastasis – a separation of the abdominal muscles (linea alba) in pregnancy.

Vaginal deliveries or the congenital state of the tissues (your collagen type), which means there is excessive distensibility of the hiatus, called ballooning, is strongly associated with prolapse and prolapse recurrence. A condition called Ehlers–Danlos Syndrome (EDS) is an inherited disorder of the connective tissue where there is excessive joint hypermobility, where the skin stretches too much and where there can be fragile tissues.[40] There are many types of connective tissues disorders which are called hypermobility spectrum disorders (HSD) and there are specific criteria which can indicate whether you may have a connective tissue disorder. Obtaining a referral to a specialist (and perhaps a geneticist) can help with appropriately managing EDS and HSD. These conditions are often underdiagnosed.

> ### Alert: Straining with your bowels can bring down prolapse
> *Repetitive straining at stool with constipation or obstructed defaecation is a common cause of prolapse in women who haven't had children as well as those who have. Ensuring correct positioning, dynamics of defaecation and the correct consistency of the stool is critical in the effective management and prevention of prolapse.*

Types of prolapse

New terminology makes it easier to understand where the prolapse is occurring. However the old names are still probably more commonly assigned to the conditions, so both have been included. Prolapse is named after the tissue or organ that has lost its support and is protruding into the vagina. The old terminology ends in *'coele'*, which means hernia or swelling.

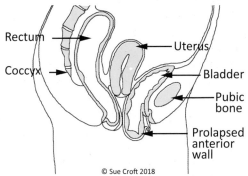

© Sue Croft 2018

*Fig 15. **Anterior wall prolapse** (Cystocoele)*

Anterior (front) wall prolapse or cystocoele (Fig 15) is due to the weakening of the vaginal walls (often from vaginal deliveries) causing the bladder to bulge into the vagina. It can often feel like a soft swelling in the front of the vagina.

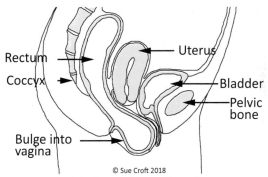

© Sue Croft 2018

*Fig 16. **Posterior wall prolapse** (Rectocoele)*

Posterior (back) wall prolapse or Rectocoele (Fig 16) is the bulging of the rectum forward into the vagina. This can feel like a soft swelling if the rectum is empty, but can feel like a hard bulge if the rectum has not been evacuated.

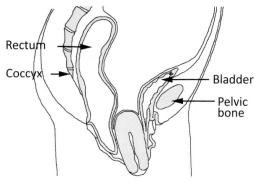

Fig 17. **Uterine Prolapse**
© Sue Croft 2018

Uterine prolapse *(Fig 17)* is a prolapse of the uterus. If the woman inserts her finger in the vagina, the cervix will be close to the opening and feel quite hard (like the tip of your nose).

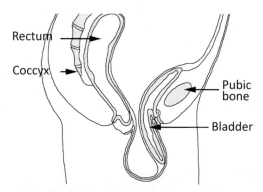

Fig 18. **Vaginal vault prolapse**
© Sue Croft 2018

Vaginal vault prolapse *(Fig 18)* Women often believe that once they have a hysterectomy (removal of the uterus) they cannot prolapse any more. However, if they have levator avulsion or significant nerve damage and if they continue to do things which first caused the prolapse of the uterus, such as straining with bowels, lifting heavy objects and gym work beyond the strength of their pelvic floor, then the top of the vaginal vault can start to fall down. This is called a vaginal vault prolapse. Major reconstructive surgery is then required to repair this.

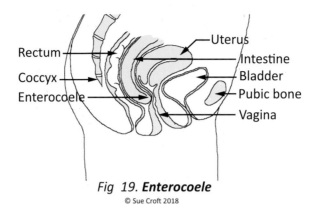

Rectum
Coccyx
Enterocoele

Uterus
Intestine
Bladder
Pubic bone
Vagina

Fig 19. **Enterocoele**
© Sue Croft 2018

Enterocoele (Fig 19) is a prolapse of the peritoneum or small bowel. This is when the peritoneal sac containing some small bowel descends into the rectovaginal space (deep behind the uterus) in the vagina. It can give the woman a heavy uncomfortable feeling and sometimes backache. An enterocoele is a marker of severe pelvic floor weakness and can often be associated with rectal prolapse. The higher the grade of rectal prolapse the more likely there will be an enterocoele present.[41] Advancing age, having had a prior hysterectomy, having other significant prolapses (anterior, uterine and posterior wall) and if you have a chronic coughs or severe physical exertion increase the likelihood of having an enterocoele. Your physiotherapist may assess you in standing with a trans-perineal ultrasound (where the ultrasound head is placed along your perineum in standing) to look for peristaltic (bowel) movements indicating there may be an enterocoele.

Urethrocoele is when the urethra protrudes into the vagina. Often this quite small prolapse causes significant concern for the woman because she can be constantly aware of the urethrocoele as it sits low, below where she can feel something constantly (*sensory zone* - above this imaginary 'line' women can't feel their prolapse, but as soon as the prolapse drops below this line, they feel something all the time, like a tampon is dislodged). So while it is a small prolapse, the women can be quite bothered by it, especially if they have looked with a mirror and are shocked by the changed 'look' of their vagina.

Remember you can still prolapse even if you have had a hysterectomy! This is called a vault prolapse.

51

Conservative strategies for prolapse

'Conservative' is the word assigned to all management strategies for pelvic floor dysfunction that are not surgical. 'Preventative' is a word that encompasses the strategies in this book as it describes an empowering action that women can undertake once they have discovered they have prolapse. As described before, there is significant evidence that the preventative strategies below can manage prolapse successfully for many years.[5,8]

- Learning how to perform a correct pelvic floor muscle contraction and undertaking a lifetime regular program of pelvic floor muscle training (PFMT).

- Engage the pelvic floor muscles at the appropriate time to prevent leakage of urine, gas or faeces (bracing or 'the knack', *page 21*).

- Remember to relax the pelvic floor muscles at the appropriate time to prevent pelvic floor muscle overactivity from developing particularly post-surgery (over-clenching to hold the surgery up).

- Always relax your abdominal and pelvic floor muscles and use the correct position and dynamics to achieve complete bladder and bowel emptying *(Chapters 4 and 6)*.

- Be pro-active with general exercising your whole life, but modify exercise programs to make them 'pelvic floor friendly' as required, to prevent unnecessary downward forces on the pelvic floor and vaginal structures if you have significant pelvic floor dysfunction or had major repair surgery.

- Be aware the activities of daily living that may increase your risk of prolapse e.g. prolonged squatting when gardening or cleaning, lifting heavy groceries or grandchildren, renovating or moving house and make sure you engage your muscles appropriately, delegate the task or get fitted with a pessary.

- Keep your weight in the moderate range as the evidence tells us that obesity increases your risk of prolapse and failure of your surgery. Losing weight as we age gets harder, but it is important to start by trying not to put anymore weight on. Getting assistance from a dietician, to not only give you the necessary education about how to lose weight, but to also make you accountable to someone by weighing in.

Increasing weight gain especially around your middle increases your risk of your surgery failing.

Prevention and watchful waiting

An important concept regarding prolapse is that of *prevention and watchful waiting*. With a Stage 1 - 2 anterior wall prolapse (cystocoele), the recommended treatment in the literature is *watchful waiting* and commencement of conservative management from a physiotherapist with a special interest in pelvic health.[42,43] Make an appointment to be assessed with a physiotherapist and learn the preventative strategies but if you cannot access anyone, the strategies are outlined in this book, should be the first line of treatment in managing mild to moderate prolapse and continued forever, even if your prolapse is significant and will ultimately require surgery.[8]

Rushing in to correct the 'anatomy' is not necessarily the best option, especially if the woman has significant muscle trauma such as avulsion. Remember if there is partial or bilateral avulsion, there can be *up to* 80% chance of failure of the surgery,[37] so maximise conservative strategies and discuss with your doctor, pelvic health physiotherapist or continence nurse practitioner the concept of trialling a pessary. *Pessaries are not just for old ladies.*

Pessaries

Pessaries are a very useful treatment strategy for managing vaginal prolapse. There are two types of pessaries - one is made of a soft medical grade silicone and may be fitted by your obstetrician, doctor, trained pelvic health physiotherapist and specially trained continence nurse. The other type is a plastic pessary which is more rigid and stays in-situ for a much longer time (can be up to 3 to 6 months) before being removed, washed and reinserted, after the vagina is checked with a speculum by your doctor.

Pessaries can be used as a short-term alternative to maximize the potential options prior to having surgery. Having the pessary inserted can give women relief from their prolapse, while they learn and perfect the necessary conservative strategies prior to their repair surgery, such as correct defaecation position and *'the knack'*.

Having a pessary fitted prior to surgery may also reveal any potential stress urinary incontinence that can be masked by a significant anterior wall prolapse (cystocoele) kinking the urethra. When there is a significant prolapse, sometimes after the surgery has been performed and the prolapse fixed up, women can be disappointed with their result post-operatively, due to newly-revealed stress incontinence. If this is discovered pre-operatively, the surgeon may decide to add a continence operation to ensure continence is maintained post-operatively.

Self managing pessaries can also be a very successful longer-term solution for prolapse self-management by the patient. The flexible pessaries can be inserted by the woman, who is taught how to self-manage the pessary with insertion and removal and cleaning it. The patient is also advised to rest the vagina from the pessary overnight. It can be used with exercise, when there is a need for prolonged standing or just to prevent the heavy dragging feeling that prolapse can cause for a woman with simple essential daily tasks, such as lifting, shopping and repetitive bending.

They are usually washed in warm water with a liquid soap (carefully follow the cleaning instructions of the manufacturer of the device, your doctor or pelvic health physiotherapist who has fitted it) and are left in for the required task or activity (e.g. running), which may only mean a few hours; or they can be left in for up to 1 to 2 days for a cube pessary; or 7 days for a ring pessary.

Follow the instructions of the manufacturer or your treating health professional for the length of time your pessary is to stay in. There are many different styles of pessaries and it is a matter of trial and error when attempting to fit one. Factors like finger dexterity, your body flexibility or your weight (particularly with a larger girth) can influence your ability to be taught how to self-manage one. Sometimes it is not possible to get a pessary to hold up which can be frustrating for the health professional attempting to fit it and of course the patient, but it is often useful to do a pessary trial to see if one will work.

Some of the significant factors for a pessary not staying in are the degree of levator avulsion, the distance of the measurement GH+PB on Valsalva *(page 17)* and /or the degree of vaginal (hiatal) ballooning. Many doctors and pelvic health physiotherapists have fitting kits (sterilized between patients) which enable you to go for a walk to see if the pessary will stay in, which is useful because they can sometimes appear to be fitting well, but then work their way down with brisker activity.

The woman is taught self-management and the pessary renewed usually yearly in accordance with the manufacturer's instructions. It is important to check for any blood, excessive discoloured or smelly vaginal discharge and remove it immediately and see your doctor. Your doctor should check your vaginal integrity yearly with a speculum if you are wearing the pessary every day. If the woman is post-menopausal then local oestrogen cream or tablet inserted in the vagina can improve the plumpness of the vagina and therefore the skin integrity to help prevent erosion of the vaginal walls from the pessary.

The complications with a pessary include: excessive vaginal discharge, bacterial vaginosis, vaginal epithelial ulceration, occult stress incontinence, fistula (where the pessary causes erosion into the bladder or rectal wall) and the forgotten pessary. [44]

A super tampon (if it can be retained) can be useful for short term reduction of a prolapse, particularly with exercise, repetitive coughing or a vomiting illness. Women are used to inserting tampons for their menstrual periods and so are familiar with the concept. It must not be left in any longer than the manufacturer recommends and *you yourself* must decide upon the use of them considering the risk of toxic shock syndrome (TSS). Take particular note of the manufacturer's instructions and precautions regarding the use of tampons. Refer to *page 39* for more on this. Using a small amount of a vaginal moisturizer (available at a pharmacy) or a water-based lubricant can be useful to counteract the drying effect from using tampons as a short-term management strategy.

More recent interesting research has looked at the value of using a specially - designed pessary post-operatively (inserted by the surgeon at operation) for the first four weeks to give early support to the operation. However, this is not routine at this point in time and while there is promising preliminary data, more research is required to establish its role in pelvic floor surgery.[45]

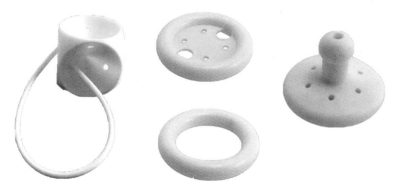

Remember pessaries are not necessarily for everyone, but they are definitely not just for old ladies!

PIPES: an acronym for pelvic health assessment

Early detection of pelvic health issues means you can often prevent worsening symptoms. I have created this acronym '**P I P E S**' to help remind doctors and patients about some simple questions that can be asked at a woman's PAP smear test.

This acronym will help you and your doctor thoroughly assess your pelvic floor dysfunction: -

- **P** stands for Prolapse (vaginal and rectal)

- **I** stands for Incontinence (urinary, faecal as well as vaginal and anal flatus)

- **P** stands for Pain (pelvic, vaginal, rectal or abdominal)

- **E** stands for Exercise (what is the pelvic floor muscle strength; general exercise levels for your cardio-vascular system; bone density; muscle fitness and sense of general well-being).

- **S** stands for Sex (any pain, low libido, lack of lubrication and even relationship issues that you may be able to discuss with your doctor).

Up until 2017, women would undergo a regular PAP smear to screen for cervical cancer (cancer of the cervix of the uterus) every two years. However recently in Australia and other countries, this has changed to be called the Cervical Screening Test (CST) which is a screening swab from the cervix for human papillomavirus (HPV) which is only necessary every five years unless there is a previous, positive test. Discuss with your doctor.

Asking your doctor to routinely check you for prolapse (and ask questions about incontinence and other pelvic health issues) at this screening test will help alert you to early signs of descent of your vaginal walls and allow you to intervene early, to avoid worsening of your prolapse. If you are aware of this vaginal descent, you will be able to see a pelvic health physiotherapist to learn the correct activation of your pelvic floor muscles; commence a program of regular pelvic floor exercises (including relaxing them at the right time); as well as reminding you to implement all the other preventative strategies listed on the previous pages.

Prevention, prevention, prevention
'A clever person solves a problem, a wise person avoids it'.
Albert Einstein

With the frequency of this test lengthening to five years as opposed to two years with the old PAP smear, the American College of Obstetrics and Gynaecology (ACOG) is still recommending annual appointments for a *well-woman examination* which fits in nicely with this concept of regular assessment of pelvic floor dysfunction. [(46)]

By opening dialogue about what is normal and what goes wrong with this most intimate area, the doctor can then refer the woman to a physiotherapist with a special interest in pelvic health, for ongoing mentoring. This connection can go on for many years - perhaps with a yearly visit to check the status of the bladder, bowel and pelvic floor function - empowering women with self–management strategies, while still being accountable to someone to ensure long-term compliance with their program.

Other important considerations

If you are breast-feeding or post-menopausal, discuss whether it is appropriate to use local oestrogen (inserted in the vagina twice-weekly) to improve vaginal tissue quality and help with prolapse management with your general practitioner or specialist doctor. Breast-feeding may suppress your monthly menstrual cycle due to high levels of prolactin - a breast-feeding hormone - competing with oestrogen and progesterone production. As time progresses following the birth, the atrophic vaginal tissues can not only impact on prolapse and incontinence, but also may cause dryness and subsequent pain with intercourse. You cease the local oestrogen when you stop breast-feeding.

Post-menopause local oestrogen also helps the vaginal tissues with lubrication for intercourse and may be necessary if any sort of supportive pessary (e.g. a ring, cube, Gelhorn or others) is to be used to help maintain any prolapse.

Vaginal mesh implant problems

Over the years, different types of **implantable mesh** have been used in vaginal prolapse repair operations. Now, after a number of years with the mesh in-situ in the vaginal wall, there have been problems with certain mesh products shrinking and/or extruding into the vaginal walls and the bladder. This has been debilitating for many women causing persistent pain, immune system problems and chronic urinary tract infections among other serious problems. Some women have not been able to be sexually active since their surgery which had a serious impact on their relationships and their sexuality.

In more recent years, there has been litigation against the companies that produced the mesh products without adequate testing prior to its sale and distribution for use in patients. This has had world-wide ramifications on the regulations regarding the use of implantable mesh in recent years, with many countries banning the use of implantable mesh in the vaginal walls to treat prolapse surgically.

If you have had transvaginal mesh implanted in your repair operation, it is important that you know from your surgeon what sort of mesh was used and immediately seek help from your surgeon if you have:

- any generalized pelvic pain.
- a sudden change in urinary frequency, urgency or urge leakage.
- chronic urinary tract infections.
- dyspareunia (pain with intercourse) for you or your partner.
- vaginal discharge with an unpleasant odour.

Get the necessary investigation to ensure the mesh is not causing damage or pain and discuss the next step with your surgeon. If you have had mesh implanted and you currently have no side effects and it is holding your prolapse well, *then do not worry.*

Summary: Management strategies for prolapse

- *Conservative measures such as pelvic health physiotherapy incorporating pelvic floor muscle training, bracing ('the knack') and lifestyle changes such as using the correct position for defaecation and modifying physical exercises if necessary. Recent research has shown that that these strategies make a significant difference in reducing prolapse symptoms, are cost effective and should be recommended as a first line of treatment.[8]*

- *Local oestrogen to help with tissue quality in an atrophic vagina (a vagina lacking oestrogen such as when breast feeding or in a post-menopausal woman). Discuss with your doctor.*

- *Pessaries can be invaluable as a short term or longer term support of pelvic organ prolapse (page 53).*

- *Surgical options if the prolapse is significant and not responding to conservative measures. A urogynaecologist, gynaecologist or colorectal surgeon will assess which operation will be most suitable for you.*

Chapter 6

Management of bowel function

It is now known that there is a strong link between poor patterns of defaecation (emptying your bowels) and problems with vaginal and rectal prolapse and bladder function. Women who are chronically constipated or who have a pattern of straining to pass a bowel motion (often learnt as young child or adopted following childbirth damage), are causing an unnecessary downward stretch on the ligaments and fascial support of their pelvic floor and the organs that the pelvic floor supports. This inability to empty effectively (even with straining) is called *obstructed defaecation* and is very common in women who have had vaginal deliveries and even nulliparous women who have difficulty coordinating relaxation of their tummy and pelvic floor to defaecate.

Signs of this are:

- Going 4 or 5 times to the toilet during the day to pass a motion and only evacuating small amounts.
- Having difficulty getting clean and having to use large amounts of toilet paper.
- Soiling some time after the passing of a bowel motion. This can be discovered when going to pass urine several hours later.
- Itching and discomfort in the anal area due to residual soiling.
- Having to lean back to pass a bowel motion.

Women can also suffer from *true slow transit constipation* where the colon may be long, slow and tortuous and motions are hard and infrequent. Often these women suffer with bloating and abdominal pain and may have even been told they suffer with irritable bowel syndrome (IBS). Even though they may in fact have these changes to their colon on colonoscopy, learning how to defaecate (pass a bowel motion) properly, can often improve their symptoms of their diagnosed IBS.

Another cause of defaecation difficulties and often a major source of pain for both men and women is when there is a *lack of coordination* between the abdominal and pelvic floor muscles known as *pelvic floor dyssynergia* (used to be also known as *anismus*). This means two muscles of the pelvic floor - the external anal sphincter and puborectalis muscles - *tighten* due to the contraction of the superficial abdominal muscles during straining. What these pelvic floor muscles should do is *relax, funnel and then open* to allow good emptying of the rectum. This poor coordination can lead to excessive straining and cause incomplete evacuation, rectal prolapse and painful anal conditions such as anal fissures and haemorrhoids.

This often starts in childhood when children are perched on a toilet without foot support or a small inner toilet seat to give them a stable base in order to evacuate. They often slump back and tightly draw in their tummies, grunt and groan and push down into their bottom. This causes the learning of a poor pattern which can lead to constipation, rectal prolapse, haemorrhoids, anal fissures and often pain, leading to stool withholding.

To avoid damage there are three components for effective defaecation:

1. Position: There is a different position of defaecation that may prevent damage to the fascia, ligaments and muscles of the pelvic floor and usually makes it easier to evacuate the stool. A common problem with many women is a sense of incomplete emptying or that the bowel motion is getting caught in a 'pocket' which is a posterior wall prolapse *(Fig 20)*. Using the position *(Fig 21)* will assist with defaecation by minimizing downward descent of your pelvic floor and help prevent damage to the nerves, ligaments and fascial structures. See *page 63*.

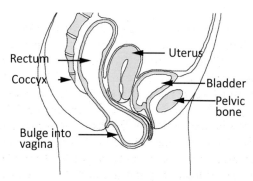

*Fig 20. **Posterior wall prolapse (Rectocoele)***
© Sue Croft 2018

2. Coordination: There is a different way of coordinating the abdominal and pelvic floor muscles to assist with opening the anal sphincter and gaining relaxation of puborectalis (one of the pelvic floor muscles). See *page 64*.

3. Stool consistency: Understanding about stool consistency facilitates easier and more complete evacuation of the rectum. The consistency is improved by obtaining adequate fibre from foods in your diet, sometimes added soluble or insoluble fibre is necessary and always adequate fluid intake. See *page 65*. Sometimes despite having good fibre intake in your diet, other products to help facilitate a 'softer' stool may be necessary.

Common bowel tests that might be performed

There are a number of tests that may be undertaken if you have bowel problems. These tests are helpful for your treating health professional to diagnose conditions and formulate a treatment plan.

Bowel Diary

A simple and a very effective diary that allows you to track the effectiveness of your bowel evacuation, of any products you are using and it also records other issues such as pain, soiling, bloating or bleeding. This information is also very useful for your treating doctor (GP, gastroenterologist or colorectal surgeon), physiotherapist or continence nurse. It can tell you the frequency of evacuation, stool size and consistency (Bristol Stool chart *page 68*) and if you add in a food diary, it can demonstrate the correlation between some foods and any bloating, pain or loose stool from foods eaten. (See *Appendix 4* for a blank form).

Ano-rectal studies

These studies reveal the resting and squeeze pressures of your internal and external anal sphincters. This test will show your values compared to the normal values and it allows your health professionals to see the status of your sphincter mechanism. Damage to the sphincters can happen from childbirth, anal surgery or repetitive banding procedures. To have the test, you are positioned on your left side with your knees bent. Anal pressure measurements (resting and squeeze) are taken by introducing a small tube into your bottom. The second part of the test involves introducing a balloon which is slowly inflated until it can be felt. You are then asked questions about the sensation of the balloon as it is filled and the balloon is also used to measure a reflex that relaxes the anal muscles. A report is produced again with normal values included to see the status of your anorectal mechanism.[47]

Endoanal ultrasound

This test will confirm the presence or absence of sphincter defects which can contribute to faecal or gas incontinence by assessing the status of the internal and external anal sphincter. Ultrasound can also be used in the assessment of recurrent and complex anal fistula and perianal sepsis.[48] A 3D/4D ultrasound can also be used to look for sphincter defects.

Track how your bowels are travelling with a simple bowel diary (Appendix 4). This allows you to see what products are working and what foods may be affecting them.

Defaecogram

A defaecogram, also known as a defaecating proctogram, is used for functional imaging of the structures used in defaecation. It is a study commonly used to demonstrate the functional problems in a person with pelvic floor dysfunction.

The defaecogram can demonstrate:
- if there is a rectocoele or posterior wall prolapse
- if there are other prolapses like a rectal prolapse, enterocoele or intussusception.
- the amount of perineal descent of the pelvic floor during defaecation
- the amount of elevation of the pelvic floor from a pelvic floor contraction
- if there is complete evacuation of the rectum
- if there is faecal soiling
- if there are signs of dyssynergia (a lack of coordination between the anal sphincter and one of the pelvic floor muscles during defaecation)

Colonic Transit study

A transit study demonstrates your bowel motility and is used in the clinical evaluation of constipation. You are given a small amount of radiotracer to drink and then go back each day for five days for a repeat scan to see how far the tracer has moved through your bowel. A simpler, inexpensive, *home* transit study is the corn test or beetroot test outlined below. This is useful to see how slow the bowel motility is because the corn shows up clearly in the stool or the bowel motion has a purple colour from the beetroot. If it is greater than 47 hours until you see the last of the corn or the purple discolouration, then this may be evidence that there may be slow transit constipation.

Corn or beetroot test:

A simple, inexpensive way to monitor your transit time is through the 'corn or beetroot test'. Firstly ensure you have had no corn or beetroot for a week; then eat a cob or bowl of corn (don't chew too well) or a moderate portion of beetroot (roasted may be easier to eat a large quantity); then have no more corn or beetroot for another week. Look at each bowel motion and note when you first see the corn or purple coloured bowel motion, and note when you last see it. If it takes longer than 47 hours to see the first corn or purple colouring and is still visible in the stool well past the 47 hours, then you may have slow transit constipation. Charcoal tablets also make the stool distinctively coloured.

Position for defaecation

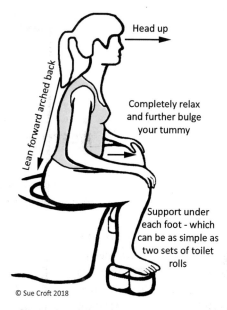

Head up →

Lean forward arched back

Completely relax and further bulge your tummy

Support under each foot - which can be as simple as two sets of toilet rolls

© Sue Croft 2018

Fig 21. Correct posture for emptying bowels

Tips for positioning for bowel evacuation: [49]

- *Keep the curve in your back as you lean forward at the hips, seated on the toilet. Lift your breasts out of the waistline. (Slumping means your breasts go down towards your waist line and changes the ano-rectal angle).*
- *Lean your hands onto your knees which are about 30 cm (12 inches) apart, whilst maintaining the curve in your back.*
- *Using a foot raise such as two inexpensive plastic wrapped rolls of toilet paper under each foot may enhance the position (see above). They should be firm and no more than 10cm (4 inches) in height. (This depends on your height and the height of the toilet - modify accordingly). Keep your feet flat on the foot raise where possible to decrease tension in your legs and pelvic floor muscles. Sometimes it may be necessary to come up on your toes, if you are at a toilet where there is no foot stool available.*
- *Your knees should be slightly higher than your hips.*

To Empty:

- Firstly, always respond to the first urge for bowels if you can. The first urge is often the best urge (except if you are post-colorectal surgery and may be getting many urges to go due to post-surgical mucosal swelling at the rectum and anus).

- If your urges are not very strong (or if children have constipation or poor bowel control), it can help to have a *'sit' for a maximum of 5 to 10 minutes,* approximately 20 to 30 minutes after a meal to capitalize on the *gastro-colic reflex.* This means that when you eat, the next amount of bowel motion is pushed along and you get an urge to go to the toilet.

- Next sit in the correct position *(Fig 21)* and then relax your tummy.

- Next *gently* further bulge your mid-tummy wall. You may find it easier to place your hand on your belly button as you do this to ensure the correct action. (For young children it is often easier to ask them to *'hissssssss'* like a snake or *'mooooo'* like a cow). This action opens and relaxes the anal sphincter. Always think about bulging your tummy *not* pushing down into your bottom.

- If you feel your pelvic floor is collapsing as you try this, then use your hand to give support at the perineal body (the area between your vagina and anus) and this will further assist with emptying of the bowel. If you have a large posterior wall prolapse (rectocoele), you can also place your finger into your vagina to help reduce the prolapse. There is also a device called a *Femmeze®* which you can use to reduce this prolapse.

- If you have significant pelvic floor descent, it is advised that you seek an individual consultation with a pelvic health physiotherapist to ensure you have the correct action and dynamics of defaecation.

- This position and muscle co-ordination is also helpful for managing painful conditions such as haemorrhoids, anal fissures, proctalgia fugax, coccydynia and pudendal neuralgia.

- It is very important to make sure the consistency of the stool is soft and easy to pass. See *page 65.*

- Children must **always** have foot support to help develop the correct pattern of defaecation and often need to aim for a slightly softer stool than an adult as long as they can still control it (Bristol Stool Type 5 see *page 68*).

Improving stool consistency

The information presented below is of a general nature and does not replace the invaluable advice that a one-on-one consultation with a dietician would provide about your individual needs.

Increasing Dietary Fibre

Fibre is the part of plant foods which we cannot digest. Fibre helps to produce softer bulky motions which move more quickly through the bowel and are easier to pass. Be aware that more fibre in your diet may increase your gas production. While 30 grams of fibre is generally recommended as a daily intake, some people find it difficult to deal with the symptoms that amount of fibre produces.

- Use more fibre-rich foods such as 2 pieces of fruit and 2½ cups a day of vegetables.[50] See a dietician if you believe you are FODMAPS sensitive *(see page 69)*. See *Appendix 1* for the website for finding a dietician.

- Be careful not to have an excessive intake of wholemeal, grainy breads, brown pastas or brown rice if you suffer with *slow transit constipation* as you may find this type of fibre constipates and bloats you more.

- High fibre snacks that contain dried fruit (prunes and apricots) may be helpful but be careful with excessive intake which may bloat you more.

- Having large amounts of unprocessed bran is not recommended as it can reduce your body's uptake of important minerals due to the presence of phytic acid.[51]

- In some people with slow transit constipation, a high residual fibre diet can 'clog' the bowel, producing discomfort and bloating. If this happens, please seek further advice from a dietician. See *Appendix 1* to help you find a dietician.

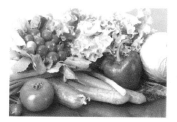
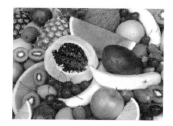

Drink plenty of water and fluids

For fibre to work properly, it is very important to drink 2 litres of fluid daily. Water is the ideal fluid as it contains no sugar. Weak cordial (watch sugar content), decaffeinated drinks, juices and milk can also be counted in your fluid intake, but water is preferable. Minimize tea and coffee as they contain caffeine which may irritate the bladder and bowel. Water-decaffeinated coffee and tea (i.e. non-chemical decaffeination process) can be used as a replacement. See *pages 35 and 36* for more fluids advice.

Soluble and insoluble fibres *(for softening and bulking your bowel motion)*

Natural and commercial soluble and insoluble fibres may assist in preventing constipation by bulking and softening the motion. Fibre is also useful to bulk up the stool when it is too loose causing faecal urgency or faecal incontinence. While it is recommended that you first use fruit and vegetables as sources of dietary fibre, there are many forms of soluble and insoluble fibre that you can use to boost your fibre intake. These fibres act on the bowel motion not the bowel wall, so they are safe to take long term. There are some examples of brands of fibres available in Australia below. Ask your doctor or pharmacist for the names of equivalent local products if you are in another country.

- *Psyllium husks (ispaghula)* are a natural fibre (2 teaspoons once or twice per day in water, yoghurt or sprinkled on cereal). Psyllium husks are gluten free but may be prone to exacerbating abdominal bloating in some people.
- *Metamucil®* (smooth texture powder or capsules) is based on psyllium husks and as such is also gluten free. The capsules are handy for travel but the dose required is up to six capsules.
- *Fibogel®* is based on ispaghula.
- *Nucolox®* is based on a mix of psyllium and maize starch, a resistant starch called starmax.
- *Benefiber®* (gluten free but based on 100% wheat dextrin) is a very user-friendly soluble fibre as it dissolves clear in water or can be added to virtually any drink without forming gel if left to sit. You can also sprinkle it on cereal and pour the milk straight on to dissolve it. It also comes in a variety of sizes including convenient travel sticks (like sugar or coffee sticks).
- *Normafibe®* is a type of insoluble fibre which produces less gas and bloating and is promoted as being useful for IBS (irritable bowel syndrome). It can be also used to bulk up loose bowel motions and as such can help with faecal incontinence. It is based on a fibre called Sterculia which is gluten free. In countries other than Australia, the equivalent product is called *'Normacol'*. Note the product called 'Normacol Plus' in Australia has a stimulant additive called *'frangula'*.

The dose and instructions for taking these products are on the containers. Please read these carefully and follow the directions especially if you are taking other medications. Do not think 'to have more is better' with fibre because if you have slow transit constipation you can get more 'clogged' if you overdo the fibre. It is always important to have an adequate fluid intake with any fibre and seek further help from a dietician if necessary. It is important to always check with your doctor regarding constipation and product use. Your doctor may prescribe different products if fibres are not working.

Other bowel products if more chronic constipation

Osmolax® and *Movicol®** are osmotic laxative bowel products based on Macrogol, which assists with drawing more water into the bowel and may be prescribed to ensure an 'easy to pass' stool if the first line of treatment of dietary modification and added fibres have not worked. *Movicol* comes in sachet form and the dose may be 1 or 2 sachets at a time with *each* sachet needing to be mixed in exactly 125 mls of water. It is also available in chocolate flavour and also half sachets (mix with only 60 mls of water). *Osmolax* has a less salty taste and is mixed with 100 to 200 mls of water. It comes in a tub with a scoop so the dose can be increased or decreased according to the stool result. There are many brands of osmotic laxatives around the world, so check with your doctor.

*Coloxyl®** tablets (50 mg or 120 mg) is another over-the-counter pharmacy medication which can be used to soften the stool.

*An adult glycerol suppository®** is helpful for evacuating difficult-to-pass motions. It is better to use one of these to assist with evacuation rather than strain. You need to take off the outer plastic casing, moisten the tip of the suppository with water, insert in the rectum and it will then take about 15 to 30 minutes to act. Initially, when first using, you are often able to keep it in longer if you lie down rather than walking around. They soften the stool and help empty the rectum (be aware it create an urgent urge to go). Sometimes you can cut them in half - enough to create a satisfactory urge to go.

A *Microlax enema®** may be necessary if the glycerol suppository hasn't been successful. These may be purchased over the counter at the pharmacy.

A useful guide called the **Bristol Stool Chart®** *(page 68),* demonstrates the desired consistency of bowel motion when using any product. Remember to discuss the appropriateness and dosages of all products mentioned above with your doctor or pharmacist.

*Product brand names vary around the world so check with your doctor or pharmacist for the equivalent product and seek advice as to whether any of these products may be helpful to your condition.

How do you judge your stool?

Adjust the amount of product you are taking so that you have types 3 or 4 on the Bristol Stool Chart shown below.

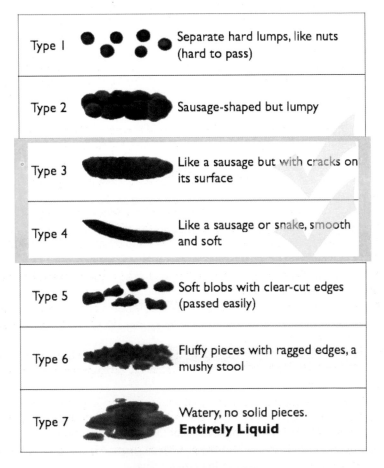

Type 1		Separate hard lumps, like nuts (hard to pass)
Type 2		Sausage-shaped but lumpy
Type 3		Like a sausage but with cracks on its surface
Type 4		Like a sausage or snake, smooth and soft
Type 5		Soft blobs with clear-cut edges (passed easily)
Type 6		Fluffy pieces with ragged edges, a mushy stool
Type 7		Watery, no solid pieces. **Entirely Liquid**

Bristol Stool Chart [52]

How to reduce problems with flatulence

Excessive gas, bloating and a lack of control of gas can be uncomfortable and embarrassing for women. Excessive gas in the sigmoid colon can also contribute to relaxation of the internal anal sphincter (the smooth involuntary muscle sphincter responsible for primary faecal control) and subsequent faecal incontinence.

There are many causes of bloating which are sometimes globally attributed to the label 'Irritable Bowel Syndrome' (IBS). Research into *'FODMAPS'* diets *(Fermentable Oligo-saccharides, Di-saccharides, Mono-saccarides* and *Polyols* which are a specific group of naturally occurring sugars) are showing benefits when managing bloating and abdominal discomfort. See a dietician if you would like more information about dietary contributions to gas production.

The following simple strategies can be helpful in dealing with gas, flatulence and faecal incontinence:

• Eat slowly and mindfully, chew your food well, avoiding bubbly drinks.

• Avoid eating too much food at a time. Everything in moderation.

• Peel skins on fruits and minimize fruits with edible skins such as grapes.

• Eat regular meals, skipping meals is more likely to increase gas production and may upset your body's routine.

• Perhaps minimize or avoid some wind-producing foods when you are *going out*, such as cabbage, brussel sprouts, cauliflower, peas, chick peas, lentils, onion, celery and nuts. Lactose in dairy can also contribute to loose stools and bloating.

• Keep a food diary to note other foods that may cause increased bloating and wind problems for you.

• Excessive intake of vitamin and mineral supplements can sometimes cause problems with gas production. Check with your doctor or dietician about what you are taking.

• Mannitol and sorbitol (found in sugar-free gum and other diet sweets) and foods high in fructose add fermentation load to the gut and can cause gas and loose stools.

• Continue to strengthen your external anal sphincter *(pages 14 and 17)* and brace these muscles with increases in intra-abdominal pressure to assist with the control of wind and faecal incontinence (soiling) forever.

• Having better bulk in the stool (e.g. with Normafibe®) will often give you better control.

• Lying on your tummy may help to shift wind if you are feeling bloated and distended.

Constipation and the subsequent retained faecal matter, can not only cause significant discomfort and heaviness, especially if the woman has a prolapse, but also can be another cause for generating considerable gas and bloating.

The strategies below not only decrease wind pain but also help move things through the bowel.

- Exercise gently to stimulate the bowel by using such exercises as the pelvic rocking and knee rolling exercises found on *page 90*.
- In standing, leaning forward onto a bench, you can also tilt your pelvis forwards and backwards .
- Walk regularly or undertake other forms of exercise. Try not to be too sedentary.
- Have a warm shower or use warm packs to help any abdominal discomfort. Women who suffer with diverticular pain (and pain from endometriosis) find this very beneficial. Be careful not to burn yourself when using a heat pack.
- *Gentle* abdominal massage to help with constipation *(Fig 29, page 91)* has been shown to give positive effects in a number of trials and is definitely worth implementing.[53] Start at the low right side of the tummy, using a circular motion as you slowly move up to waist level, move across above the belly button and down the left side.

Faecal Incontinence

Faecal incontinence is soul destroying. *'The negative impact and embarrassment related to bowel accidents is lasting and causes ongoing anxiety about the possibility of a future occurrence.'* (Christine Norton 2013) So, it is the unpredictability of these accidents that cause almost as much angst and anxiety as the faecal incontinence episodes themselves.

Faecal incontinence has many causes but can be due to: a weak internal and external anal sphincter which can be damaged by tears or nerve damage sustained with childbirth; ageing; radiation; neurological conditions; surgery; straining at stool; faecal impaction (where watery faecal matter moves around the hard stool or there may be a stretched rectum with poorer sensation); stools that are too loose (which can be caused by your diet, by parasites or bowel conditions such as irritable bowel syndrome, colitis or Crohn's Disease) amongst others.

'The negative impact and embarrassment related to bowel accidents is lasting and causes ongoing anxiety about the possibility of a future occurrence.' (Christine Norton 2013)

Treatment strategies for faecal incontinence

- Using products that manipulate the stool consistency (the *'too loose'* stool) by bulking (Normafibe, Benefiber).
- Ensuring that the rectum (and any rectocoele or posterior wall prolapse) is evacuating completely, by using the correct position and dynamics for defaecation (*pages 63 and 64*). There is a useful saying to help you understand this: *'An empty vessel doesn't leak'*. What this means is - if you sit properly, using the correct dynamics and empty the rectum completely (the vessel), there is less likely to be any soiling.
- Performing *'the knack' (page 21)* prior to any increases in intra-abdominal pressure (IAP) also helps to close off the voluntary sphincter of the anus (EAS) and helps to contain the stool and gas. Prior to coughing, sneezing, bending or lifting, tighten your vagina and particularly your anus to help contain the gas or stool.
- Research shows that using a medication helps to slow bowel motility and improve the tone of the internal anal sphincter. Discuss this with your doctor or pharmacist.
- Managing your diet well to decrease gas producing foods that may reflexively cause relaxation of the internal anal sphincter (the involuntary sphincter). It is useful to see a dietician to help you with this.

Summary points

- Avoid straining and try not to defer the urge to go with your bowels.

- Repeated straining at stool can cause pelvic floor descent, prolapse, haemorrhoids, anal fissures, anorectal pain and potentially damage any gynaecological or colorectal repair surgery.

- Don't be afraid to use a glycerol suppository (or if very constipated you may need a Microlax Enema®) to assist evacuation and therefore avoid the damaging effects of straining.

- Allow sufficient time to go to the toilet, not rushing, but do not sit on the toilet for too long if there is no action.

- Use unperfumed flushable wipes (for the final wipe only) if you have any faecal incontinence or if you suffer with haemorrhoids or anal fissures - available from the 'toilet roll' aisle in your supermarket in purse size and large pack. Use in moderation for the sake of the environment.

7 Chapter
Managing persistent pelvic pain

Over the years since the first edition of this book was published, it has become increasingly apparent that tenderness in the pelvic floor muscles can become a problem for many women. There are many reasons for this.

As a society, we encourage women to sit tall and discreetly, with their legs crossed (so their adductor or inner thigh muscles are tight) and with a flat tummy. This posture increases tension in all these muscles.

Also, those who have prolapse, urinary incontinence or faecal incontinence can have increased tension or cramping in the muscles (and potentially pelvic pain) as a result of just *'hanging on for grim death'* with their pelvic floor muscles. Constipation and straining at stool can also cause pelvic pain (called *proctalgia fugax*) due to traction of the nerves (the pudendal nerve see *page 73*) to the area. Women after any gynaecological or colorectal repair surgery can also be fearful that their surgery may fail if they don't clench their pelvic floor muscles all the time. Anal pain can also occur after colorectal repair surgery.

Ongoing, un-resolving low back pain, being posturally correct (i.e. never slumping) and trying to aim for strong *'core stability'* can also result in your abdominal and back muscles never being relaxed which can increase your pain. Pelvic pain can be associated with endometriosis with tender areas in the pelvic floor muscles contributing to this persistent pelvic pain condition. Finally chronic emotional stress and anxiety can result in over-activation of the pelvic floor muscles.

For all these conditions therefore, it is important to have *a moderate approach to tightening your abdominal wall and pelvic floor muscles.* For some women it is like walking a tight-rope - balancing between tightening their muscles enough for better bladder, bowel, pelvic floor control and post-operatively to obtain a good surgical outcome and *not excessively tightening them* which could potentially cause a spiral into persistent chronic pain.

Persistent pelvic pain can lead to sexual dysfunction at any time through a woman's life. Painful intercourse (dyspareunia) can significantly affect the quality of life of the woman and affect her ability to have a fulfilling relationship. Younger women who have never had children, can develop persistent pain associated with the pelvic region. Their symptoms include: tightness in their pelvic floor muscles (*levator myalgia or overactive pelvic floor muscles*); never been able to have penile penetration during sexual relations; difficulty inserting a tampon; voiding dysfunction (unable to empty their bladder completely); extreme pain with a PAP smear when the speculum is inserted or discomfort when wearing tight clothing.

These symptoms describe a condition known as *provoked vulvodynia*. It has been associated with chronic thrush, but may also have no apparent cause. It is important to always have a diagnosed swab confirming thrush rather than self-medicating from the pharmacy because you are itchy or have a discharge in the vaginal region.

Pudendal neuralgia (PN) has symptoms of burning, stabbing or shooting pains related to the distribution of the pudendal nerve. The pudendal nerve arises from S2-S4 nerve roots carrying motor (movement), sensory (sensation) and autonomic (not under our voluntary control) fibres. It feeds to most of the pelvic floor muscles, the perineum, the clitoris, the last part of the urethra, the anus and rectum.

A diagnosis of PN is based on an extensive history taking from the patient and their signs and symptoms rather than a lot of medical tests.[54] Patients often have significant hyperalgesia (increased sensitivity to mild painful stimuli), allodynia (pain in response to nonpainful stimuli), and paraesthesia (sensation of tingling or numbness).[55]

Another very distressing condition that can occur is called *bladder pain syndrome* (BPS), also known as *painful bladder syndrome* (PBS), or *interstitial cystitis* (IC). This condition causes women to suffer extreme frequency, urgency and pain associated with their bladder as though they have a urinary tract infection, but on testing, the urine is usually always clear. As patients with BPS try to hold on constantly against these repeated urges to go, they can also develop tightness in their pelvic floor muscles.

It is important for women to seek help from a pelvic health physiotherapist if they have *any* persistent pelvic pain. Whilst some of the conditions can appear suddenly and can be of unknown origin, advances are being made all the time in our understanding of how to manage persistent pain in general and *persistent pelvic pain* specifically. For this group of patients it is very important to teach specific pelvic floor muscle training which concentrates on *relaxation* of the pelvic floor muscles rather than tightening them. This is called *pelvic floor down-training*.

Always get a high vaginal swab to check for thrush from your doctor rather than self-medicating with over-the-counter thrush medication from the pharmacy.

Some treatment strategies for persistent pelvic pain

Treatment of persistent pelvic pain is never quick and easy and can be frustrating for both the patient and their physiotherapist. No physiotherapist likes to see their patients suffering, and patience and resilience is needed from both parties. Some of the strategies that could be used to help with these conditions may include:

- *Specific education regarding the physiology of pain*. When physiotherapists and your other health professionals start to teach you about the 'newer understanding of pain' - *that it is due to central pain mechanisms - meaning the brain decides whether there is going to be pain or not* - the patient will often have the feeling that their medical carer or therapist might think that it is all in their patient's head! This is not the case. The science of pain is well-researched and has changed rapidly in the past two decades and every day we are learning more about the physiology of pain.[56] Pain is very complex but entirely treatable. Pain education is the cornerstone of treatment, once any red flags (other pathology that may be the culprit) have been eliminated. The patient needs to understand that the treatment can be slow and requires them to *keep moving muscles and exercise* when their instinct might tell them otherwise. An excellent text called *'Explain Pain'* by David Butler and Lorimer Moseley *(Appendix 1)* simply explains the complexity of persistent pain, often using metaphors, stories and very simple language to make the science easier to understand. They have now produced a workbook for patients which is recommended to all readers called *The Protectometer (Appendix 1)*. It allows you to work through your own pain story and apply their suggestions to your own life experiences.

- *Relaxation therapy*: Learning how to gently release or relax the abdominal muscles and pelvic floor muscles at different times through the day. Think of the pelvic floor as though it were a lift or elevator and when there is stress and anxiety, then the pelvic floor muscles - the elevator - may be sitting at the third floor. By relaxing your abdominal muscles - letting your belly go soft and consciously letting go with the pelvic floor muscles, you can bring the elevator down to the ground floor or the basement.

At different times we must know how to relax all the muscles of the body, but particularly the pelvic floor muscles.

Your pelvic floor muscles can be like a barometer of your stress and anxiety and so checking through the day if you are unconsciously *turning them on* and making an effort to consciously *let them go* is important, particularly when you are experiencing significant life stress.

- *Music therapy* can be conducive to effective relaxation. Make a play list of music that you enjoy, but tends to be gentle and relaxing. If heavy metal rock is your go-to genre to help decrease anxiety, then use whatever works for you. Listen to the music while you do a full body scan (see below).

- *'Sit like a man'* - the image you conjure up when you think how a man sits is: leaning back and somewhat slumped, with legs exaggeratedly apart and belly 'off' and relaxed. In our society women are encouraged to always sit tall *'like a lady'* with their legs crossed and to always have a flat tummy. If you never let go of your muscles, sometimes this can lead to increased tone in all the muscles around the abdominal, pelvic and hip region and can exacerbate pelvic pain, with increased tension in your pelvic floor muscles.

- *Do a full body scan* assessing the status of all your muscles, what is tight and switched on? What is in a nice relaxed state? Work through each muscle group letting them go. See the check list below.

Body scan checklist:

☐ *Relax your scalp*
☐ *Make sure you aren't frowning*
☐ *Slightly open your mouth so you aren't clenching your jaw*
☐ *Drop your shoulders*
☐ *Do a gentle upper chest breath (bra breath)*
☐ *Now gradually bring your breathing down into your tummy*
☐ *Place your hand over your belly and feel it rise as you breathe in and drop away as you breathe out*
☐ *Let your tummy muscles relax*
☐ *Let your pelvic floor muscles switch off*
☐ *Let your adductors (inner thighs) flop out*
☐ *Back to another tummy breath*

- *Breath awareness* is very important in managing pelvic pain. We know that mindful breathing can lower your heart rate and help manage anxiety more effectively. Effective breathing can help stop you invoking a panic reaction which increases the chance of a tightening response in your pelvic floor muscles.

When you breathe in the upper part of your chest (apical breathing) you tend to breathe faster and shallower, giving you a low level of carbon dioxide in your blood which can make you feel dizzy, leave you feeling breathless and increase your anxiety. Doing mindful breathing (belly breaths) can be life-changing for any anxiety you are suffering.

Start with a *'bra breath'* - this means have a breath in and feel the side of your chest around your bra region expand gently and out at the sides and then let it go as you breathe out. Do this four times and then move down to do some *tummy or belly breaths.* Place your hand on your tummy and as you breathe in, your tummy should rise up under your hand and as you breathe out, your tummy should drop back down. Take your time to practise this. If you own a Fitbit®, you will often observe a significant drop in your heart rate as you do belly breaths.

- *Specific massage* of the tender points in the pelvic floor muscles using vaginal dilators or a therapeutic wand, just as you would massage tight neck muscles if they had spasm and tightness in them. Your pelvic health physiotherapist will teach you how to use the dilators or a therapeutic wand and give you a home program to follow (*Chapter 10*). The dilators or wand also decrease the *fear factor* which has heightened over the months or years - a fear that the vagina is very *'fragile'*. What is helpful is to think of the vagina as *'robust'* and strong - it delivers babies and can tolerate vigorous intercourse when there is good arousal and no pain. The adductor muscles (the inner thighs) are often tightly clenched and guarding the entrance to the vagina, so if you attempt to use the dilators, you could be massaging pelvic floor muscles which are being tightly held and this will naturally be painful. Keep your inner thighs relaxed and well supported and do stretches of them regularly *(Figs 22 and 23).* Supporting your legs on pillows to the side will be helpful also.

- Some women also find learning about *mindfulness* and *meditation strategies* can be very helpful for managing persistent pelvic pain.

- *Advice regarding sexual intercourse* such as ensuring adequate attention is given to arousal, utilising more 'outercourse', use of non-irritating lubricants, use of non-latex condoms and positional advice can all be useful *(Chapter 15).*

- S*pecific medication for pain:* Your physiotherapist may suggest you see your GP or specialist for a prescription which can be very helpful with this type of pain. It is an older antidepressant medication - not because the doctor thinks you are depressed (although some women may suffer with depression with this debilitating condition) - but that this older style of medication given in quite low doses has been shown to help pelvic pain by decreasing the messages from the periphery (the vagina, the pelvis, the bladder - whatever is painful) through the spinal cord and on to the brain.

- *Exercise advice*: *'Motion is lotion', 'nerves need to slide and glide'*[56] - nerves love to move and these word images are helpful visualisations for self-treating persistent pelvic pain. Pace and grade your return to movement (or sexual activity), so that the gradual re-introduction of this activity does not lead to a flare up of pain. The message of moving and exercising is very important, but some women do excessive numbers of abdominal strengthening exercises such as sit-ups, double leg lifts and a full plank and therefore give themselves intensely strong abdominal muscles. This means they can find it difficult to ever *let go* with their abdominal wall and this not only causes a *winding up* of the pelvic floor muscles and pudendal nerve that feeds to this area, but can also cause voiding dysfunction. The non-relaxing pelvic floor leads to emptying difficulties of the bladder, causing women to have a slow stream, or perhaps a start-stop-start flow rate and subsequent residual urine left in the bladder after attempting to urinate. This can contribute to chronic urinary tract infections. (See *Page 34* for the position for emptying your bladder).

- Using the positions below will assist with keeping nerves gliding and sliding and moving within their sheaths and can help with persistent pelvic pain. Check with your pelvic health physiotherapist about any modifications necessary if you have had gynaecological or colorectal surgery or have prolapse *(Figs 23 and 23 below)*.

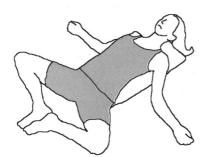

Fig 22. Lying butterfly pose
© Sue Croft 2018

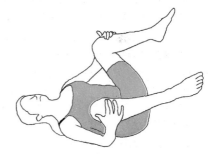

Fig 23. Modified baby pose
© Sue Croft 2018

Remember

- Treat acute pain early and appropriately including post-op pain.

- Do not over-grip your muscles furiously post-op, trying to hold the surgery up, as this can lead to pain developing.

- Always balance all tightening of your pelvic floor and abdominal muscles with relaxation.

- Education is one of the cornerstones of the management of persistent pain. Pain science is well researched and adapts well to treating pelvic and vaginal pain.

- Even reading some of this pain education can start to improve your pain.

- It is the always the brain which decides whether something hurts.[57]

- The amount of pain you experience does not necessarily relate to the amount of tissue damage you have.[57]

- With persistent pain, when you are hurting, it doesn't always mean you are damaging yourself.

- The brain has 'plasticity' which allows us to modify our response to pain. This brain plasticity got you into this pain situation, but the brain plasticity can also get you out of it.

- Pacing and graded exposure to movement, exercise and sexual intercourse is important in the recovery from persistent pain.[57]

- Sometimes you may be encouraged to reduce high levels of pain relief to reduce persistent pain as the opioids can actually prolong your pain by making you more sensitive to pain over time. This is called hyperalgesia and makes these medications generally less effective for chronic pain, as you progress to need higher and higher doses. Some animal studies have even shown that opioids can set off immune signals in the spinal cord which amplify the pain.[58] Your pelvic health physiotherapist and other health care professionals will help you through the process.

- There are many blogs written on managing persistent pain. Just google 'Sue Croft Blog Persistent pain resources in one location' and there are many links to pain resources within that one blog.

- Relapses can happen but you have the knowledge to put in place a program to return you back to your pain-free state.

- Don't ever give up!

Chapter 8

Pre-operative physiotherapy expectations

As with any surgery, whether it be a knee ligament reconstruction, a total hip replacement or back surgery, it is always advantageous to have a pre-operative work up prior to that surgery to ensure you are well-educated about the upcoming surgery, have optimised muscle strength and therefore enhanced the chances of a good result...*and the same applies to any gynaecological or colorectal repair operation.* A well-informed, well-educated, well-prepared patient is always going to have a less traumatic hospital stay and a better recovery than one who has had little work up.

Pre-op Routine

- *Ideally patients can be sent to a physiotherapist with a special interest and training in pelvic health approximately three months prior to their surgery. If the surgery is deemed to be more urgent than that, then it is still useful for the patient to try to have an individual consultation with the physiotherapist prior to surgery. Some private practices and public hospitals have group pre-operative education classes for their patients which are also very beneficial.*

- *This allows:*
  - *pre-operative assessment of bladder and bowel function including a pre-op bladder diary (Appendices 2 and 3) and a bowel diary (Appendix 4).*
  - *pre-operative assessment of the pelvic floor muscles to see if there is correct muscle activation and assess for strength, potential nerve damage or muscle avulsion, endurance and importantly, breath control.*
  - *you to discuss any hip or back pain issues which may need to be reported to the surgeon (i.e. care with stirrups and handling on and off the operating table).*

- *The patient can then commence an appropriate muscle strengthening program for the pelvic floor prior to the operation.*

- *There is also an opportunity to retrain poor bladder habits, teach 'the knack' and train the habit of 'bracing' and teach the correct positions for bladder and bowel emptying.*

What does an individual appointment with a pelvic health physiotherapist potentially involve?

- *Extensive education* about normal and abnormal bladder and bowel function – regardless of what your condition is or what operation you are having. This is often supported by handouts or brochures. This ensures that you do not continue with bad habits which may lead to other problems in the future.

- *An internal muscle examination.* This is a routine occurrence by *specially trained* physiotherapists to assess your muscle strength and teach you the correct action and interaction of the pelvic floor muscles and deep abdominal muscles. This is invaluable in giving you feedback about your pelvic floor muscles which sometimes give poor sensory feedback to you due to childbirth damage, previous gynaecological surgery or radiation treatment. *Informed consent* will be obtained prior to this internal examination.

- If you are seeing a physiotherapist in rural areas where there is no specialist pelvic health physiotherapists available, you may be able to have the local physiotherapist use a 'real-time' ultrasound machine to check the activation of your pelvic floor muscles.

- A pre-operative before and after-void bladder scan may be performed. This involves an ultrasound of your full bladder and then you will be asked to urinate and then re-scanned to check how well you have emptied the bladder and to check for any residual.

- You will be asked to perform a 2 day bladder diary *(Appendix 2 and Appendix 3)* and while this might seem a bother when trying to find 2 days when you are home, it is an important assessment tool for the physiotherapist or doctor to thoroughly assess bladder function, particularly pre-operatively.

- A routine of preventative exercises for circulation, deep breathing and some exercises for post-operative back or wind pain *(see pages 86 and 91)*. These have been positioned in the post-operative section of this book for ease of access whilst using this book in hospital.

A summary of a physiotherapy pre-operative home program

- Pelvic floor muscle training (PFMT) which includes learning the importance of relaxing the pelvic floor muscles as well as strengthening them.

- 'Pelvic floor friendly' abdominal muscle exercises.

- Practise *'the knack'* and habit of bracing with all increases in intra-abdominal pressure.

- Teaching how to get in and out of bed after the surgery so it can be practised at home.

- Implement the new position for voiding (emptying the bladder) by completely relaxing the low tummy and pelvic floor. Don't strain to empty.

- Bladder retraining (if necessary) using the urge control techniques to achieve 350 to 500 mls bladder capacity. Don't overfill your bladder if you have any retention post-operatively. Know if you are emptying completely (by ultrasound) and if you're not emptying completely, aim for closer to 350 mls rather than 500 mls voided.

- Decrease or eliminate caffeinated drinks, maintain adequate hydration but don't overdrink.

- Use the correct position and dynamics for defaecation. Make good changes to your diet to ensure a soft, easy-to-pass stool.

- You will be taught specific strategies if you have pelvic pain issues.

- Practise belly breathing *(pages 75 and 76)* in the leadup to the surgery to control any anxiety that may be present.

When patients have had long term problems with their bladder and bowel function it is often difficult to let go of old habits and implement some of the changes. *Sir Francis Bacon* summed it up nicely with the following:

"Remember the greatest obstacle to progress is the belief that no progress is possible!"

The correct mindset - plan well!

The secret to a comfortable and successful post-operative experience once you come home from hospital is being well prepared in advance, have firm guidelines as to what you can and cannot do and **stick to them.**

It is not a chance to clean up the spare room, repaint the lounge room or 'shop till you drop'. Get a good supply of books, record lots of your favourite television programs and have a list of letters / emails to write or phone calls to make that you have been meaning to do for ages and take it easy in your recovery phase. The following guidelines are really meant for major gynaecological or colorectal repair surgery or if you have had a hysterectomy, rather than more minor stress incontinence surgery (such as a mid-urethral sling)

- Rest is important. Having major repair surgery can be exhausting and you will be surprised how much you need to sleep in those early weeks at home.

- Shopping before the operation to ensure adequate provisions and perhaps doing online shopping when the initial supplies run out, so they can be delivered not just to the door, but right into the kitchen.

- Depending on the help you have at home, meals cooked and frozen beforehand are great but there are also many businesses which provide frozen meals delivered to your door for a reasonable cost considering you don't have to shop to buy the ingredients and don't have to stand and prepare them for lengthy periods of time.

- Train your partner and/or children to pitch in with cooking and house-hold chores and tell them what you can and cannot do in the immediate post-op period. If the housework isn't happening put on a pair of blinkers and ignore the mess. It just isn't worth the risk of damage to maintain a pristine house at this time.

- It is better to pay for some cleaning services once a fortnight rather than risking your repair surgery and trying to do it yourself. Avoid cleaning the bathroom or doing the vacuuming for six weeks if you have had major repair surgery and have weak pelvic floor muscles. Whilst gardening may be relaxing for you, it involves repetitive bending, sometimes squatting and often heavy lifting or digging, so the heavier gardening tasks are best avoided in the first 12 weeks post-operatively.

- Your surgeon will advise you as to when you can commence driving again after your operation. Adhere strictly to his / her advice as you may affect your car insurance if you drive before you should and subsequently have an accident in the car.

- Once you have had the operation, you should avoid shopping for at least a fortnight and not push a loaded shopping trolley for at least 6 weeks. Take a partner, older child or friend with you where possible to do the heavy work of lifting the shopping for at least 6 weeks.

- Again it is not a time to catch up on dinner parties – (especially not ones at your place). You may find it quite uncomfortable to even sit for lengthy periods of time due to perineal pain and some colorectal repairs can mean your anal sphincter region is very painful. You do not want to be standing and cooking for long periods of time either.

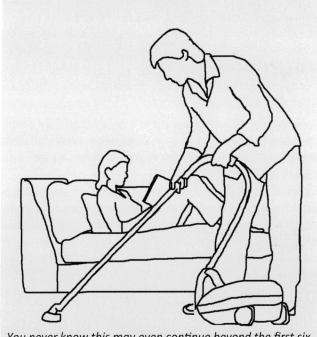

You never know this may even continue beyond the first six weeks!

The immediate post-operative period

You have woken up following your surgery and hopefully you have no nausea or vomiting and initially at least, very little pain. Below are some important points to allow your hospital stay to be a success.

- Having adequate early pain management is very important post-op, as it allows you to move more easily and therefore prevent complications such as deep vein thrombosis and chest infections and it hastens your departure from hospital.

- It is important to communicate effectively and honestly with the nursing staff and your surgeon regarding your pain – there are no bravery awards given out for refusing pain relief! This is also important for preventing persistent pain from developing.

- If you have any nausea or vomiting ensure you ask for medication to help this (anti-emetics) and if vomiting, place your hand over your vaginal pad to give perineal support (around the vaginal or anal region) to your new operation.

- It is important to minimise visitors in hospital as they can be tiring and you need to rest and recover for your discharge home. Don't sit for long periods of time as this encourages swelling to develop or persist post-op.

- Eat simply and lightly – choose options with a higher fibre content to help get your bowels moving post-operatively and avoid caffeinated drinks which may irritate your bladder. If you have no bladder issues, some caffeine can help your bowels.

- Make sure your catheter is strapped to your leg to ensure it doesn't get tugged or caught in the bed sheets and cause urethral discomfort. Once your catheter is removed be aware of your fluid intake and how long it is between your voids (wees) so you *don't overfill your bladder.* Communicate early and clearly with your nurse regarding this as well. See the section on catheter care on *page 85*.

- Never strain to pass urine or a bowel motion. The vaginal pack can be quite big and may cause extra bowel pressure. Do not strain thinking there is stool to shift. This may cause haemorrhoids and damage your surgery. Never hold in wind - you will feel very uncomfortable because your bloated belly will increase your pain and discomfort and it is an important sign that your bowels are moving well post-op. It will help you pass the wind if you place your hand over your vaginal pad at the front through to just before the anus and give some perineal support.

Catheter care

Often following major gynaecological or colorectal repair surgery or simply a hysterectomy you will have a catheter inserted to rest the bladder and assist with its complete draining. Some helpful hints regarding catheter care will minimise discomfort and prevent long-term damage to the bladder.

- Always ensure the catheter is strapped to your leg to stop urethral irritation from the catheter getting tugged accidentally or caught up in the bed clothes.

- When going for a walk always make sure the catheter bag is detached from the bed and either you or the nurse are holding it, or it is attached to your drip pole. The catheter is held in the bladder with a small inflated balloon and if you walk away from the bed with it still attached to the bed, there may be significant damage to the urethra if it is dragged out.

- It is not uncommon for the bladder to be slow to get going again after repair surgery. Sometimes the catheter will have to be re-inserted if you are unable to void (wee) once the doctor gives permission for it to be removed. The nursing staff are very vigilant about ensuring you do not overfill your bladder once the catheter is removed. (Remember the correct storage volume of the bladder is 350 to 500 mls). Long term bladder damage can occur if your bladder very significantly over-fills post-op.

- If it takes a bit longer for voiding (urinating) to get going due to swelling post-operatively, you may need to learn *self-catheterising* before you go home. Do not panic about this as the nursing staff will help you with it. A bladder scan is often performed quite a number of times to check your residual urine volume. You will need to get your residuals (the amount you have left behind) down to 100 to 150 mls (depending on your surgeon) before you are allowed to cease self-catheterising.

- Once you go home from hospital, if you have a sudden change in urinary symptoms such as frequency, urgency and urge leakage always check with your surgeon or doctor regarding the possibility of having a urinary tract infection. There does not need to be pain on voiding, blood in the urine or a feeling of passing razor blades when voiding for you to have an infection. Urine should be clear (as opposed to cloudy) and not have a strong odour. These characteristics may also indicate infection.

In hospital: post-operative physiotherapy routine

The following exercise routines are designed to prevent chest and circulation complications. You will sometimes be fitted with compression stockings (TEDS) and given injections to prevent deep vein thrombosis in your legs, but the following routines of deep breathing and circulatory exercises will further prevent serious post-operative complications.

1. Deep breathing exercises

To help prevent post-operative chest complications, take a long deep breath to expand and fill the bases of your lungs, pause then relax as you breathe out. Repeat 10 times every hour.

2. Prepare and engage your pelvic floor muscles when moving (Fig 24)

Immediately post-op remember to prepare prior to moving to protect your surgery. Breathe in and out normally, then gently engage your pelvic floor muscles gently prior to moving (bracing, *'the knack'*). Turn on these muscles before any cough and sneeze especially. *(See Fig 26 for more detail.)*

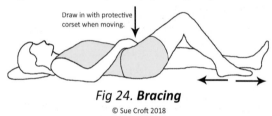

Draw in with protective corset when moving.

Fig 24. **Bracing**
© Sue Croft 2018

Caution:

You can turn on your pelvic floor muscles to support and move as mentioned above, but ask for surgeon's specific advice about recommencing pelvic floor exercises post-operatively. Each surgeon has their own protocol and currently there is no evidence supporting any recommendation regarding the timing of commencement of pelvic floor exercises.

3. Protect when you cough (Fig 25)

If you have an abdominal incision or port holes from laparoscopic surgery then it is important to minimize abdominal pain by tightening your pelvic floor muscles and gently slide your knees up one at a time. This takes the stretch off any abdominal wounds. Keep the pelvic floor contracted and support any wounds with your hands and forearms as you cough strongly to clear any secretions. A pillow or a towel supporting the wound is also helpful for decreasing pain from any abdominal incision or portholes from laparoscopic surgery.

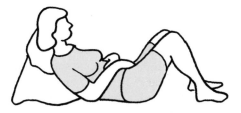

*Fig 25. **Protect when you cough***
© Sue Croft 2018

If you have had vaginal repair or colorectal surgery, *place your hand over your vaginal pad* and gently contract your pelvic floor to prevent violent descent of your pelvic floor when coughing or if you vomit post-op. It is a good idea to check with your anesthetist or surgeon that you are prescribed a medication called an 'antiemetic' - a drug which helps nausea and vomiting.

Advice:

Cough strongly if you have any secretions to clear and prevent a chest infection or pneumonia developing - but ensure you brace and use hand support beforehand.

4. Circulation Exercises

The following exercises are important in conjunction with TEDS stockings to assist in prevention of deep vein thrombosis (DVTs) and should be done half to one hourly. Do 5 to 10 at a time.

- Tighten your pelvic floor muscles and gently slide your legs up and down *one at a time* .
- Pump your ankles up and down vigorously to help with the muscle pump and the return of the blood to the heart.
- Tighten your thigh muscles, hold for 5 seconds and then let go.
- Squeeze your buttock muscles, hold for 5 seconds and let go.

5. Breathing Exercises Using a Triflow®

If you have a pre-existing chest complaint you may be given a breathing device (Triflow®) by your hospital physiotherapist to help you take deeper breaths regularly and prevent post-op basal atelectasis (collapse of the small airways in the base of your lungs).

6. How to move further up the bed

- Have the head of the bed fairly flat. Engage your pelvic floor muscles. Bend your knees up one at a time until your heels are closer to your bottom.

- Dig your elbows and heels into bed and then making sure your pelvic floor is engaged, push up the bed.

- *Do not* use the monkey ring above the bed (if there is one) as it strains your abdomen and surgery site and increases intra-abdominal pressure pushing down on your repair operation.

7. How to get out of bed when lying on your back (Fig 26)

- You are going to roll your whole body and legs together as a single unit (log roll), towards the side of the bed *where your catheter, drip and drain are attached.* Continue to breathe throughout this whole process.

- Firstly, while lying on your back, tighten your pelvic floor muscles and draw your knees up one at a time. Make sure you have enough room between your body and the edge of the bed to roll without falling out. Maintain the pelvic floor contraction and roll onto your side keeping your shoulders, hips and bent legs in line.

- If you have rolled to the left side for example, dig your left elbow into the bed and push through your right hand, gently lowering your legs over the edge of the bed. Keep your ankles and feet moving to stop you feeling dizzy after sitting up. *Breathe, tighten your pelvic floor and keep your knees bent.* It is important to practise this to each side, prior to your operation, so when you are in hospital you are confident about getting out from either side.

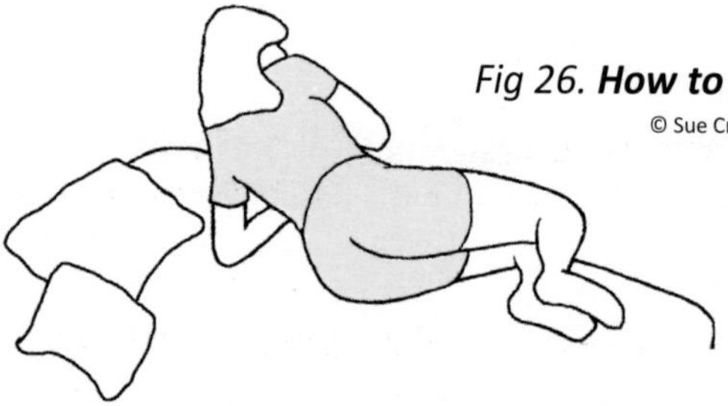

Fig 26. **How to get out of bed**
© Sue Croft 2018

Hint:
Sometimes after rolling onto the same elbow all the time, your elbow can become quite tender. It helps to vary the side you are getting in and out of bed, once your drip, drain and catheter are removed. Some patients have found wearing a long sleeve or a cut off sock over their elbow can act like a protector and cushions the elbow.

8. Mobilising

When first going from lying to sitting, to help with any dizziness from the position change, keep breathing, look out the window (if possible) and pump your ankles up and down. Make sure you keep breathing low and slow - do not hyperventilate or this may cause you to feel faint.

When going from sit to stand once you have sat up at the edge of the bed, to minimise pain and ensure your operation is protected, think of the saying *'nose over your toes'* and as you stand vertically, this will stop you placing excessive strain on your abdominal wound or vaginal repair.

> ### Hint:
> *Nose over your toes when going from sit to stand.*

When going for your first walk, make sure that you have adequate pain relief administered 30 minutes before the walk. It is important to have a nurse or physiotherapist with you for that first walk, to ensure you are moving safely and in case you feel faint.

> ### Hint:
> *Ensure the catheter is attached to you not the bed when going for a walk.*

Always remember to have that *catheter attached to you,* not the bed when mobilising. If you walk away forgetting it is still attached, there will be significant urethral trauma as the balloon is pulled down the urethra.

> ### Hint:
> *Recline to rest rather than sitting up all day in bed or on a chair.*

As the days continue post-operatively you will be feeling more comfortable and mobilise more easily, but always move through your side, engaging your muscles to support your repair when getting into and out of bed. *Recline to rest* rather than sitting for prolonged periods of time in hospital to minimize swelling in the perineal region (around the vaginal/colorectal repair).

9. Exercises for helping with post-op low back pain and wind discomfort

Often after laparoscopic surgery or vaginal repair surgery (performed with the patient in stirrups), there can be uncomfortable wind pain, hip or low back pain for a short time. The following exercises are helpful in relieving this discomfort. If you have back pain that persists, ask to see the physiotherapist in hospital.

(a) Pelvic Rocking (Fig 27)

Have the bed fairly flat. Gently contract your pelvic floor and bend one knee up at a time, so that both knees are bent. Slowly flatten your back into the bed by rocking your pelvis back, allowing your tummy to gently draw in. This should give relief not cause any pain. Repeat 5 times.

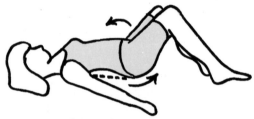

Fig 27. **Pelvic rocking** © Sue Croft 2018

(b) Knee rolling (Fig 28)

Have the bed fairly flat. Lie on your back with your knees bent up. Gently contract your pelvic floor and slowly and gently rock the lower half of your body (knees and hips) half way to one side, then to the other. Only go as far as comfort allows – do not strain your wound at all. This should not cause any pain. Repeat 5 times to each side.

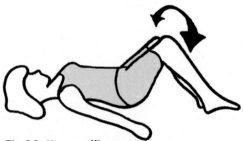

Fig 28. **Knee rolling** © Sue Croft 2018

10. Pelvic Floor and Bowel Function:

Wait for your doctor's advice about recommencing pelvic floor exercises post-op. However, make sure you engage your pelvic floor muscles with all increases in intra-abdominal pressure, to protect the surgery *('the knack')*.

Below are some strategies to *reduce wind pain* (which can be quite debilitating post-operatively).

- Exercise gently to stimulate the bowel such as the previously mentioned pelvic rocking and knee rolling exercises; in standing, you can also tilt your pelvis forwards and backwards whilst leaning forward onto a bench; take regular short walks.
- Have a warm shower or use warm packs to help.
- *Gentle* abdominal massage *(Fig 29)* can also help. Start at the low right side of the tummy, using a *gentle* circular motion as you slowly move up to waist level, move across above the belly button and down the left side, but not if there is too much abdominal discomfort from laparoscopic port holes or from an abdominal incision.

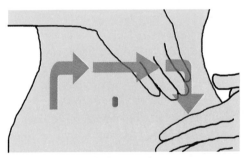

*Fig 29. **Abdominal massage***
© Sue Croft 2018

11. When emptying your bowels (page 63):

- *Never strain, never lean back and push down into your vagina and bottom to evacuate the bowel.*
- Keep the curve in your back as you lean forwards at the hips. Hands onto your knees and look ahead. Use a low footstool (such as toilet rolls) one under each foot with knees apart (unless there is a very low toilet in the hospital).
- Allow the abdomen to first relax and with your hand over your belly button, further bulge your tummy forward. This action opens the anus, creating a funnel, to help let the bowel motion out *(page 63)*. You may also place your other hand over the vaginal pad to help support the perineum.

- Choose food from the menu with good fibre content. Include extra fresh fruit, salads and fluids. Osmotic laxatives such as Movicol® (each sachet must be mixed in *exactly 125 mls water*) or Osmolax® (less salty taste and mixed with 100 to 200 mls of water) may be routinely given in hospital and can be continued at home for a few weeks or until your doctor says to cease. If good bowel motions are established you can then use added fibre instead of the osmotic laxative in the form of Benefiber®, Metamucil® or Normafibe®. These are Australian brands of fibre. In other countries check with your doctor or pharmacist for equivalent brands.
- You are often required to have passed a bowel motion before you are allowed home. If you are unable to evacuate you may need to be given a glycerol suppository® or Microlax enema® to assist with the first motion to avoid straining.
- After some colorectal surgeries, the bowel motions can be loose and frequent. This takes time to settle and can be as long as 6 weeks before the frequency settles down. Applying a barrier zinc cream (such as Sudocrem® in Australia) to the anal region can be helpful if there is anal discomfort from frequent wiping.

12. Further recovery once home:
Continue with your exercises at home and never strain – whether it be with your bowels, lifting or housework. Remember, think 12 weeks, not 6 weeks, as the recovery time post repair surgery, when maximal 'good' fibrosis, healing and strengthening of the repair surgery has occurred.

- Pelvic floor strengthening: Re-commence pelvic floor exercises once the doctor has given permission. *This depends on the protocol of your surgeon.* Always check with your own doctor. For many it could possibly be around six weeks for major surgery, but may be earlier if you have had a simple stress incontinence operation such as a mid-urethral sling.
- If you have had colorectal surgery and have anal pain or spasm, then only do a few anal sphincter exercises and ensure that you relax the muscles completely once you have ceased the exercise. Anal pain can be due to anal sphincter spasm from over-gripping.
- If you have had any urinary retention postoperatively, wait until normal voiding has established before recommencing pelvic floor exercises. See *page 10* for instructions regarding pelvic floor exercises. Always take your time to perform them (no rushing) and always relax your tummy and pelvic floor muscles completely between exercises.

10

Home recovery

The early days 1-6 weeks

To help with longevity of your operation, here are some guidelines to follow for the first six weeks. The old saying *'there is no gain without pain'* definitely does not apply in this situation. If you feel discomfort after the activity you have undertaken, then *slow down, shorten the distance you have walked or halve the time on the exercise.* Please ask your doctor or treating physiotherapist any questions if you are unsure about the advice here and always follow your surgeon's written and verbal advice.

Guidelines for first 6 weeks (major repair surgery):

- Walking and gentle exercise is important in these early weeks. When you start walking again after surgery, always walk in ever-increasing circles around the neighbourhood with your house at the centre, so you are never too far away from home (short distances initially and then build up). If you get any drag, ache or heaviness, then you can return home quickly.

- Keep your bowels formed but soft and avoid any straining forever.

- Minimize prolonged sitting (especially at the computer) as this may cause swelling. It may also exacerbate any buttock pain that may be present due to some operations which have a suture attachment to a ligament in the buttock or exacerbate swelling around the rectum and anus with colorectal surgery (in that region).

- Minimize repetitive bending in the early weeks. Buy a *'picker-upper'* which is available at big hardware stores.

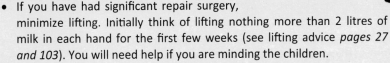
'Picker upper'

- Minimize prolonged standing. Build up slowly, pacing yourself.

- If you have had significant repair surgery, minimize lifting. Initially think of lifting nothing more than 2 litres of milk in each hand for the first few weeks (see lifting advice *pages 27 and 103*). You will need help if you are minding the children.

Weeks seven to twelve are equally important to allow the surgery to gain full strength. This will assist you to achieve an excellent outcome with your surgery. As previously mentioned, the failure rate for gynaecological repair surgery in the literature can be up to 30% with normal pelvic floor musculature and can be as high as 80% if there is significant levator avulsion (muscle trauma) and vaginal ballooning. Think about the risk factors and ask yourself— *'what are my pelvic floor muscles like?'* and be sure to switch them on prior to lifting weights and wait until 12 weeks for higher impact exercise to avoid early failure of the surgery.

Guidelines to observe for weeks 7 to 12:

- Avoid *any* straining with bowels. Continue to eat healthily; use a bowel product (fibre or osmotic laxative) and/or a glycerol suppository as required or as directed by your doctor to assist with evacuation.
- Perform daily pelvic floor exercises.
- *Still minimize repetitive bending,* especially if you have had major repair surgery.
- You can gradually increase the length of your walk but listen to your body. If you feel any drag, heaviness or ache, stop and rest!
- Still *avoid lifting* wherever possible. If you mind young children you must still try to avoid lifting them.
- Pace yourself with return to household chores. Vacuum or clean only one or two rooms per day.
- No squatting when gardening. It is preferable to kneel on a soft kneeling pad to weed the garden. Pace yourself and do half an hour the first time and see if there is any drag or ache the next day. If you are feeling good then gradually extend the length of time in the garden. Avoid digging holes with a spade and avoid moving heavy pot plants. Remember, good fibrosis of the surgical repair occurs around 12 weeks when collagen reaches 80% of its tensile strength.[8]
- Take someone with you to help with the shopping or continue to shop online and get the order delivered.

Advice for after 12 weeks

Once 12 weeks has passed, it is important to enjoy the freedom and comfort that your repair surgery presents you while still following the principles relevant to *your pelvic floor* and *your individual health issues* to ensure longevity with your operation (*Chapter 12*).

Guidelines for return to exercise for after 12 weeks :

- *Avoid* sit-ups, double leg lifts, a full push-up or a full plank. Always engage your pelvic floor muscles first and try a push-up or plank from the knees. Assess for downward vaginal pressure as you perform these exercises. See *Chapter 11* for a list of *'pelvic floor friendly'* abdominal exercises to do at the gym or at home.

- *Avoid* lifting heavy weights until you have been assessed by your pelvic health physiotherapist and always discuss any weight restrictions with your surgeon. Read the evidence regarding lifting weights in *Chapter 12.*

- *Avoid* leg press machines at gyms (where you are in a compressed position with your feet on a plate and pushing the heavy weights with your legs.) See *Chapter 13.*

- *Avoid* rowing machines if you have had major repair surgery and any other gym equipment that excessively increases your intra-abdominal pressure until you have sought advice from your pelvic health physiotherapist .

- *Assess* exercises in pilates and yoga classes and adjust applying *'pelvic floor friendly'* principles. See *Chapter 11.*

- *Avoid* high impact classes and always keep one foot on the ground (rather than jumping) when exercising. Good options include walking on a treadmill, exercise bike (low resistance), cross trainer and seated upper limb machines with the lowest weights, doing repetitions until the muscles you are exercising are fatigued.

Caution:

When coughing, sneezing or vomiting. you must where possible use *hand support or sit on the edge of a table or chair* to stop the tremendous forces which push downwards onto your pelvic floor. Take care particularly if you have hay fever, the flu, a vomiting bug, a flare up of asthma, a chronic cough such as in bronchiectasis or chronic bronchitis.

11 Chapter

'Pelvic floor friendly' exercises

Now you are at week 12 post-operatively, it is important to have a list of abdominal strengthening exercises to use if attending a gym or just doing a home exercise program. There is good evidence that if women are strong there will be better health outcomes into old age. However, some exercises such as full sit-up exercises and double leg lift manoeuvres increase your intra-abdominal pressure and if you have weak pelvic floor muscles, vaginal or rectal prolapse and especially if you have had gynaecological or colorectal repair surgery, it is better to modify these exercises.

Thinking about ways to modify exercises will reduce the number of women who experience pelvic floor dysfunction, particularly prolapse, as a result of exercise regimes that are *beyond the strength of their pelvic floor*.

When doing the following exercises start gently and ensure there is not excessive in-drawing at the waist or that your chest and ribs are not puffed up as this increases downward pressure. Keep breathing through the exercises as breath-holding increases intra-abdominal pressure.

With the following exercises you are to concentrate on *engaging the pelvic floor muscles*, as well as what your legs are doing. All these basic exercises can be performed in bed or on a floor mat. Start by doing 1 or 2 repetitions of all the exercises and then gradually build up, assessing how you feel the next day and always breathing and maintaining control with the pelvic floor.

Pelvic floor friendly abdominal exercises

1. Transversus abdominis and pelvic floor:

Lie on your back, knees bent up, gently contract your low tummy and pelvic floor muscles Hold for 5 seconds while continuing to breathe See also *pages 10 and 19*. To help you do this correctly, imagine you are doing up a zipper on your jeans and you are drawing your pubic hairline in gently as you do up the zipper. It is important to continue to breathe through the exercise and relax after you have finished.

Finish your exercises with abdominal and pelvic floor relaxation

2. Pelvic rocking (Fig 30)

Lie on your back, gently contract your pelvic floor and bend one knee up at a time, so that both knees are bent. Slowly flatten your back into the bed by rocking your pelvis back, allowing your tummy to gently draw in. Repeat 3 to 5 times. Breathe and relax after this set.

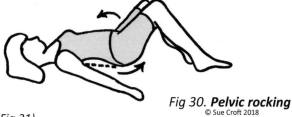

Fig 30. **Pelvic rocking**
© Sue Croft 2018

3. Knee rolling (Fig 31)

Lie on your back with your knees bent up. Gently contract your pelvic floor and slowly and gently rock the lower half of your body (knees and hips) half way to one side, then to the other. Repeat 3 to 5 times to each side. Breathe and relax after this set.

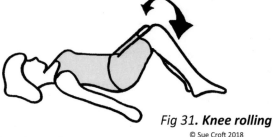

Fig 31. **Knee rolling**
© Sue Croft 2018

4. Bent knee fall out (Fig 32)

Lie on your back, with both knees bent up; gently contract your pelvic floor; slowly lower your bent right leg to the side and slowly bring back upright again. Aim to stop your pelvis from rocking from side to side. Repeat with the other leg. Do for 5 to 10 times. Breathe and relax after this set.

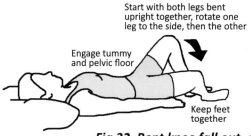

Start with both legs bent upright together, rotate one leg to the side, then the other

Engage tummy and pelvic floor

Keep feet together

Fig 32. **Bent knee fall out** © Sue Croft 2018

5. Modified straight leg raise *(Figs 33A & 33B)*

Lie on your back, knees bent up, gently contract your pelvic floor while continuing to breathe. Keeping your pelvis steady, draw your right leg to the chest and then straighten your leg out, holding the straight leg about 8cms (3 inches) off the bed/floor for a count of 3 and then go back to starting position. Repeat 5 to 10 times. As this becomes easier, do this exercise as described above but increase the number of straight leg raises to firstly 3 and then 5 if no discomfort. Remember always concentrate on the gentle tightening of your lower tummy and pelvic floor. Breathe and relax after this set.

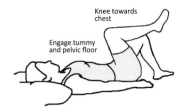
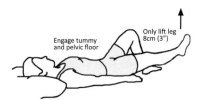

Fig 33A. **Modified straight leg raise - movement 1**
© Sue Croft 2018

Fig 33B. **Modified straight leg raise - movement 2**
© Sue Croft 2018

6. Lying abdominal exercise *(Fig 34)*

Lie on your back as usual, gently tighten your pelvic floor. Holding a *light* weight (you could even use a can of baked beans) with both hands. Slowly raise and lower the weight in a controlled manner, first from the line of the abdomen up to the shoulder line (see diagram) and then from the shoulder to back over your head. Start with 2 or 3 and build up slowly to 10 in each direction. Breathe and relax after this set. Increase the weight as you get stronger.

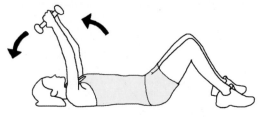

Fig 34. **Dumbbell floor press**
© Sue Croft 2018

98

7. Bridging (Fig 35)

Lie on your back, with your knees bent up, gently contract your pelvic floor while continuing to breathe; then tighten your gluteal (buttock) muscles and then slowly lift your bottom up 10 cm (4 inches) and hold for 3 seconds, then slowly lower down. Repeat 5 to 10 times. Breathe and relax after this set. As you become stronger, lift and lower without touching the bed 3 times and then rest for 3 seconds and repeat. Do 5 to 10 times.

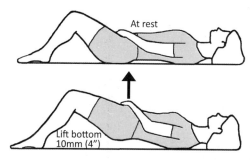

*Fig 35. **Bridging exercise***
© Sue Croft 2018

8. Modified clam (Fig 36)

Lie on your side, with your knees bent and feet together, gently tighten your pelvic floor. Keeping your feet together, lift your top leg 8 cm (3 inches) off the other leg. Do not roll your pelvis backwards as you lift. Hold for 3 seconds and slowly lower down. Repeat with the other leg. Do 5 to 10 times. If performed correctly, this is also a good exercise for the pelvic floor. Breathe and relax after this set.

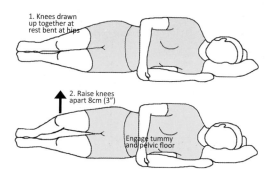

Fig 36. 'Clam' leg lift exercise
© Sue Croft 2018

9. Pelvic rocking in 4 point kneeling *(Fig 37)*

This is also a great postural stretch and is known as a 'cat curl'. On all fours, hands under shoulders, knees under hips, maintain your lumbar curve, gently contract your pelvic floor and then stretch your back up, while dropping your head down - hold for 5 seconds then return back to the start position. Breathe and relax after this set. Repeat 5 to 10 times.

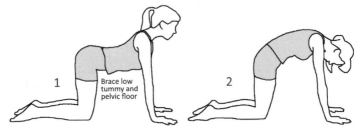

Fig 37. **Pelvic rocking in 4 point kneeling**
© Sue Croft 2018

10. Balance, abdominal and coordination exercises *(Fig 38)*

On all fours, hands under your shoulders, knees under your hips, maintain your lumbar curve. With your head in a neutral position, gently contract your pelvic floor, lift your right arm out in front, hold for 3 to 5 seconds. Repeat with your left arm. Repeat 5 times each arm.

Back to all fours and gently contract your pelvic floor muscles and lift your right leg straight out behind you and hold steadily for 3 to 5 seconds and lower. Repeat with the left leg. Start by performing 2 exercises with each limb and then as you get stronger build up to 5 and then 10.

Then, when feeling good strength (no shaking or dropping your pelvis) and quite controlled in each exercise you can lift your right arm and left leg together, hold for 3 to 5 seconds and then repeat with left arm and right leg. Breathe and relax after this set. Repeat 5 times each side.

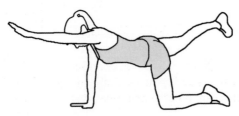

Fig 38. **Abdominal and balance exercise**
© Sue Croft 2018

11. Ball exercises (Fig 39)

Balance work on a gym ball is great for your abdominal muscles. Make sure your hips and knees are at right angles and your pelvic floor muscles are gently contracted. Start by holding your upper limbs at 90° and then lower and raise back to start position trying to keep the ball steady. Do 2 or 3 to start with and increase the number daily. Another ball exercise is to try lifting one leg 3cm (1 inch) off the ball and lowering back down again without your pelvis shifting or the ball rolling. Avoid sit ups on a ball. Breathe and relax after this set.

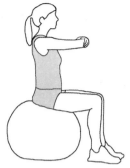

*Fig 39. **Exercise ball sit***
© Sue Croft 2018

12. Wall squat (Fig 40)

Standing with your back against a wall, your feet are approximately 30 cm (12 inches) away from the wall. Most importantly, your heels should be under your knees so your lower legs are vertical. Gently contract your pelvic floor, and slowly slide your back down the wall 8cm (3 inches) and hold the position for about 5 to 10 seconds and then slide back up again. As the weeks go by you can increase the length of hold to strengthen your central muscles and your thighs. Do not go down to 90°. *Do not do this exercise if you have knee pain.* You can use a Swiss ball behind your back as well. Breathe and relax after this set.

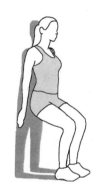

*Fig 40. **Wall squat***
© Sue Croft 2018

13. Standing Leg lift (Fig 41)

Standing, holding a chair lightly for balance. Gently draw in your pelvic floor slowly lifting your right knee to hip level and then slowly lower down. Do this 5 times slowly and carefully and repeat with the other leg. Breathe and relax after this set.

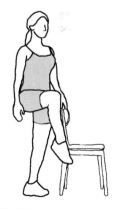

*Fig 41. **Standing leg lift***
© Sue Croft 2018

14. Forward lunge *(Fig 42)*

Many women enquire about lunges. Housework often involves bending to lower levels and the lunge is a good leg strengthening exercise. Contract your pelvic floor first and then lower down into the lunge. Breathe and relax after this set. Keep the legs apart with a narrower base if your pelvic floor is weak. Repeat 5 to 10 times.

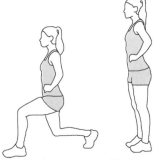

Fig 42. **Forward lunge**
© Sue Croft 2018

15. Heel drops *(Fig 43)*

Hands on the back of a chair initially, (with shoes on) come up on your toes and drop your heels into the floor. Do 5 and build to 10. You can also do without chair support – place hands on hips, knees slightly bent, come up onto your toes and again 'bang' your heels into the floor. This is a good exercise for bone density.

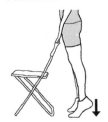

Fig 43. **Heel drops**
© Sue Croft 2018

16. Mini squat *(Fig 44)*

Stand tall with feet straight ahead and hands on hips. Gently tighten pelvic floor and slowly bend to 45 to 60 degrees at hips / knee. Incline trunk slightly forward, maintaining a gentle curve in the lower back. Squeeze gluts to come up - pushing through heels. Bring your trunk to upright and relax gluts and pelvic floor. Repeat 5 to 10 times.

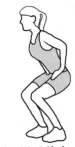

Fig 44. **Mini squat**
© Sue Croft 2018

17. Wall push ups *(Fig 45)*

Start facing the wall with feet 50cm (20 inches) away from the wall. Hands on wall just below shoulder height. Bend your elbows lowering your chest onto the wall. Draw shoulder blades back and down as you go. Keep shoulders back as you push back out. Repeat 10 times.

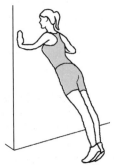

Fig 45. **Wall push**
© Sue Croft 2018

The evidence about activity restrictions

Before discussing a return to physical exercise in the next chapter, it is important to look at some of the evolving evidence about lifting restrictions following gynaecological repair surgery. Note that the factors which cause recurrence of rectal prolapse also relate to excessive intra-abdominal pressure generation due to straining with bowels and excessive weight-lifting. Over the years many of the stated weight or activity restrictions have been inconsistent, have not necessarily been based on randomized control trials and often based on the experience of the surgeon and 'common sense'. However, this is changing dramatically with many research studies being undertaken. It will be interesting to observe developments of this subject in coming years.

In this chapter, the small number of studies currently published have been presented to outline the complexity of how to advise a woman to return to exercise or what weight lifting restrictions should be given to her, if any. One important message is that you, the patient, should be individually assessed and advised depending particularly on the findings of *your* pelvic floor, *your* individual risk factors for recurrence and what *your* exercise wishes may be.

The first six weeks post-operatively can be frustrating because of the necessary limitations that need to be applied to ensure healing of the repair surgery. Fortunately the fact that there can still be significant pain is in itself a natural '*limiter*' on what you attempt to do. Unfortunately at this point in time, there is no Level 1 evidence about lifting restrictions or physical activity restrictions post-operatively.[59,60] However, if there is 80% of wound strength attained by 12 weeks[9], then it seems logical to wait until that time before commencing more vigorous exercise to maximise the potential of a lasting repair.

When trying to work out advice to give women pre and post-operatively to ensure they do not suffer recurrence of the prolapse, it is important to not restrict women so much that they are *fearful about doing anything* and stop exercising altogether. If they stop exercising, it may then increase their risk of other health issues developing such as cardio-vascular problems, bone and muscle strength deterioration and mental health issues.

The evidence does show that some activities of daily living (ADLs) have quite high intra-abdominal pressures compared to some activities that may be normally restricted post-op, such as not lifting more than 5 kg for the first six weeks. For example, getting out of a chair (rising from sit to stand) has the same intra-abdominal pressure generated as lifting 6 kilos off the floor, which is why it is so important to engage your pelvic floor muscles prior to going from sit to stand.[27] Interestingly, research has shown that lifting 0 kg (no weight) using the squat manoeuvre generated more intra-abdominal pressure (IAP) than lifting 10 kg off a counter or receiving 15 kg into outstretched arms.[27] It has also been shown that some common actions undertaken, such as going straight up from lying to sitting and when getting out of bed, have greater increases in IAP than lifting 5 kg in weight.[59] This is why you are advised to engage your pelvic floor muscles and roll through your side to get in and out of bed in hospital and once you are home or when exercising at Pilates or Yoga.

However, Nygaard et al (2013) reported that the ranges of IAP during specific activities are large and such pressures during activities commonly restricted (such as a curl up) and not restricted (such as going from sit to stand) after surgery overlap considerably. Measured the same way and doing the same standardized activity, the IAP in one woman may be very low and another very high.[60,61]

Further research undertaken on the effects of walking speeds and carrying techniques on IAP in women has shown that *the double arm hang*, which is the technique used in the exercise the farmer's walk (an exercise at the gym or like carrying your groceries in from the car), had the lowest IAP when compared to other lifting techniques, including lifting up and carrying weight in a back pack, indicating that the position of the weight above the centre of mass may contribute to IAP.[62,63]

Also higher IAPs were noted in other awkward lift and carry situations such as the 'front carry' which is what is necessary when lifting and carrying a load of washing Therefore, walking with a weight in each hand at a gym may generate less pressure on your surgery than carrying the same weight of wet washing to the line.

Finally, there is a 2017 article by Margaret Mueller which compares *liberal* with *restricted* exercise advice after reconstructive surgery. She notes at 3 months there was no difference between the two groups on the anatomical position of the prolapse, and the patients in the liberal exercise group were more satisfied on reassessment. However, while these patients were only followed up across 3 months post-operatively in the research article, there is currently ongoing research with this group to see how they are faring two years after surgery (communication with the author).[64]

So you can see this subject can be complex and, taking into account the factors we *do* know that cause recurrence of the prolapse post-operatively may help you to work out a program with your treating physiotherapist that will ensure your exercise does not contribute to failure of your surgery.

What we do know:
Factors affecting vaginal prolapse repair surgery outcomes

The articles referenced in this section relate to gynaecological repair surgery but there are also issues with recurrent rectal prolapse in colorectal surgery.

The recurrence rate for rectal prolapse repair is higher in the perineal approach (Delorme's procedure) compared with the abdominal approach (abdominal rectopexy) but the age of the patient may determine which approach is chosen by the surgeon. The perineal approach (via the rectum) is better tolerated by the elderly, but is prone to failure in younger age groups.[65] Assessing risk of return to exercise and potentially modifying exercise prescription is important for patients having colorectal repair surgery also.

Vaginal prolapse repairs have a high failure rate: The incidence in the literature of failure of any gynaecological repair surgery (such as with an anterior/ posterior repair and sacrospinous colpopexy (SSC) can be up to 30% with a rate of 10% to 20%, requiring repeat surgery[64,65] and if there is levator avulsion present (partial, complete on one side or bilateral avulsion) and ballooning of the hiatus (*page 16)* there is a risk of recurrence of *up to 80%*.[37]

The severity of the prolapse at the time of operation: Prolapse that is graded at grade 3 or 4, meaning that the prolapse is more advanced preoperatively, is associated with a higher risk of recurrence postoperatively.[66]

The state of the patient's pelvic floor affects the outcome: The Modified Oxford Scale (MOS) is a grading system used by physiotherapists and doctors assessing the pelvic floor strength of the patient. If the muscles are graded as a MOS of 0 to 3, there is between a 35 to 45% risk of recurrent prolapse.[66,67] Other articles go on to state that prolapse recurrence following surgery is a common complaint with the state of the patient's pelvic floor muscle seeming to be the strongest determinant.[68]

Other factors predisposing to failure of the surgery (particularly for the anterior compartment or the front wall) are: younger age, parity (the number of children), family history of prolapse, previous hysterectomy, enlarged genital hiatus with hiatal ballooning, collagen type (connective tissue diseases), BMI and habit of breath holding when exercising (significantly increases IAP).[69,70]

The state of your pelvic floor influences your risk of prolapse recurrence

105

What to do post-operatively about lifting and return to exercise? Factors affecting prolapse repair surgery outcomes

At this point in time there is no clear Level 1 evidence about maximum weights to lift and exercise restrictions to apply post-operatively. Rather than applying a blanket ban on lots of different types of exercise, when it comes to deciding what to do and when to do it (if ever), perhaps it could come down to a number of factors that will determine how careful and how restrictive you should be. Discuss the following with your surgeon and your physiotherapist.

- What is the severity of your prolapse at the time of operation?
- What is the state of your pelvic floor? Get checked by your local pelvic health physiotherapist.
  - Get an accurate idea of your pelvic floor muscle strength.
  - Do you have any muscle trauma (levator avulsion-one side, both sides)?
  - What is your GH+PB on valsalva? *(Risk of prolapse: Normal Less than 7cms; Mild 7 to 8cms; Moderate 8 to 9cms; Severe 9 to 10cms; Very severe >10cms. 8.5cms and above could indicate levator avulsion.)*[21]
- Are you overweight?
- Do you have an increased girth measurement?
- Do you have any connective tissue diseases?
- What are the specific guidelines from your surgeon regarding exercise restrictions? Always clearly ask your surgeon's advice and write it down so you don't forget.

Activity and exercise restrictions

If you have had repair surgery, with significant prolapse at the time of operation, or levator avulsion, or weak pelvic floor muscles, or a collagen disorder (EDS, HSD see *page 48*) or you are overweight, then:
- Avoid high impact jumping, keep one foot on the ground. Do heel drops *(page 102)* to help maintain bone density.
- Avoid sit-ups, double leg lifts and the full plank.
- Engage your pelvic floor muscles before increases in IAP.
- Keep exercising your whole life for good health.
- Where possible review regularly (yearly) with your pelvic health physiotherapist to monitor and progress your exercise and pelvic floor program and to check that your surgery is holding up.

Chapter 13

Return to exercise

Specific gym advice

The gym is a great place to get some of your exercise. It has a constant temperature when there are extremes of weather and there is often an opportunity to establish friendships and a sense of community in some studios or gyms. This is important because health recommendations for exercise for women include 150 minutes of moderate intensity exercise and two or more days of muscle strengthening activities per week.[71] Maintaining good total body muscle strength through a variety of exercise is important for women throughout their life-stages to improve balance, maintain a healthy weight and stave off the effects of osteoporosis. Exercise also makes your mind and body feel good.

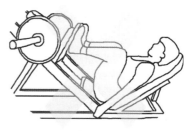

Assess the risk

However, at home or in the gym it is important to assess what is the load being placed on your pelvic floor and therefore your surgical repair, before you tackle any new exercise offered to you by a personal trainer, an exercise DVD, a pilates instructor or yoga teacher. Make sure you tell them you have had pelvic floor repair surgery. You have invested a lot of time and money in your operation and if you have those risk factors *(pages 105 and 106)* which increase the chance of recurrence of the prolapse following surgery, then assess the exercise and if necessary ask your instructor to modify it. The message is clear though, keep exercising following your operation.

Healthy bones and osteoporosis prevention

The gym is a place where you can address issues such as maintaining good *bone mineral density (BMD)*. Current recommendations for the prevention of osteoporosis with ageing in women includes regular, high-intensity, weight-bearing exercise.[72] Exercises shown to be helpful include weight-lifting, resistance training and high impact exercises such as boxing and jumping. However, the intra-abdominal pressures generated precludes jumping if you have high risk factors i.e. levator avulsion, weak pelvic floor muscles, poor tissue quality. Heel drops on *page 102* will give a decent 'pounding' effect through the long bones. Dead lifts with lighter weights (increase slowly) and seated weight machines address osteoporosis exercise requirements to help the muscles provide mechanical forces on bone resulting in maintenance or gain of bone mass.

107

Specific sports advice

Keeping active your whole life is one of the most important things you can do to live a long and healthy life. Having strong muscles and bones, good reflexes and balance not only ensures better quality of life and is important for falls prevention, but also allows endorphins to be released and stress hormones (adrenaline and cortisol) to be better managed. However, if you have had gynaecological or colorectal repair surgery, have pelvic floor weakness or residual prolapse, then some sports can place strain on your surgery and may cause it to fail.

If you play high impact sports such as basketball, netball or love jogging or running it is important to discuss your return to those activities with your surgeon and pelvic health physiotherapist. If possible, make an appointment with a pelvic health physiotherapist for advice about your post-operative sport options. Remember if your pelvic floor has been assessed and if you have significant levator avulsion and therefore an enlarged hiatus and poor pelvic floor support, then your risk is higher for prolapse recurrence and you may need to modify some exercise choices.

Walking:

Brisk walking is a friendly option for your pelvic floor. With time, introduce some hills to increase your aerobic capacity and increase the distance as it becomes easier for you. There is no hurry, you have the rest of your life to regain any lost fitness. As time progresses hiking adds challenges as well as nurturing good memories.

Running, netball or basketball

These are all high impact activities. It is important to discuss with your surgeon if and when you should go back. If you have had continence surgery such as a mid-urethral sling, the recovery time and restrictions following this type of surgery are different and less restrictive. Often the continence surgery has been performed to *allow you to continue playing your sport.*

However, if you have had prolapse repair surgery you will need to be assessed and factors such as your pelvic floor muscle strength and genital hiatus (the distensibility of your vagina) will determine whether you should resume running or playing your sport. If you have been assessed to play, initially only play one or two quarters and build up slowly over the weeks. Check with your surgeon whether a pessary maybe a useful adjunct when playing a high impact sport.

Cycling (is a lower BMD activity)

Cycling (both stationary and road) is a safer option for exercise when you have pelvic floor issues. The seat is supportive but if you have a significant prolapse or have had gynaecological repair surgery then take care when riding up steep hills where the effort is greater. Standing up to pedal puts considerable downward forces on your pelvic floor. If you have had recent surgery then make sure you keep to flat roads and paths until well healed. Using a well-padded seat cover will help with buttock discomfort. Be aware of downward vaginal pressures with high intensity cycling and high resistance on the bike in gym 'spin' classes.

Swimming (is a lower BMD activity)

Swimming is a good option if you have pelvic floor problems but is for muscle strength and flexibility rather than improving bone density. The water provides buoyancy and lowers impact. Check with your surgeon about when you may return to swimming especially if you have any vaginal discharge (otherwise wait until at least 6 weeks post-op). Flutter kicking lengths of the pool, 'deep water walking' forwards and backwards, aqua aerobics (no double leg lifts or any high resistance exercises) and swimming lengths builds up strength and endurance.

Rowing, Outrigger Canoeing, Kayaking

These water sports have gained immense popularity recently and they can all place a heavy load on the pelvic floor. Even if you are very careful about bracing, the lifting of the heavy boats will place a downward force on your operation. Check with your doctor or treating pelvic health physiotherapist.

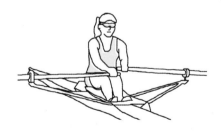

Following significant repair surgery, pay attention and stop if the exercise you are doing causes excessive downward pressure into the vagina. The operation may fail if you overdo certain exercises.

14 Chapter

Travelling

If you have a holiday planned following your surgery it always wise to wait until at least 6 weeks post-op for the following reasons. Check with your surgeon for advice.

- *Deep Vein Thrombosis (DVT)* - Anyone who has had surgery is at higher risk of developing a deep vein thrombosis (blood clot) post-operatively. Wait a minimum of 6 weeks and possibly 12 weeks for more major surgery, especially if it is a long haul flight.

- *Heavy lifting* - Travelling interstate and particularly overseas involves lifting heavy baggage which may place unwanted strain on the recent repair surgery. The longer time frame since the operation, the better chance of the *good fibrosis* to form and assist with holding the surgery in a good position. Always engage your pelvic floor muscles carefully when lifting luggage.

- *Constipation* - Many women find that travel often causes constipation and if you strain to pass a bowel motion then you will risk damage to your operation. Therefore the longer the time post-op, the stronger the surgery is likely to be and always manage your bowels well.

- *Travel tummy and bowel bugs* - anyone can get a 'travel bug' and have violent vomiting and diarrhoea which will place great strain on your operation.

To help plan a successful holiday following surgery, there is a travel checklist with ideas which will be helpful in dealing with these situations. The checklist is on *page 112* which you can photocopy and tick off prior to departing to make sure you have thought of everything when packing.

Travel checklist:

☑ *Travel light* – when packing be ruthless, remembering that once you have had gynae /colorectal repair surgery minimizing heavy lifting is important.

☑ *Always have a 'pull-along' bag with wheels* and if travelling with someone, ask them to lift the bags for you. If you have to do it, always remember to brace prior to lifting the bags.

Travel checklist continued:

☑ *Pack airline travel socks* or alternatively if you have your calf TEDS from hospital you may like to put those on under your loose long pants.

☑ *Keep your legs and ankles moving on the plane.* Every 30 minutes *while awake* pump your ankles up and down, do foot circling, tighten your thigh muscles & squeeze your buttock muscles. Walk the aisles. Adhere to airline recommendations regarding prevention of deep vein thrombosis (DVT's).

☑ *Talk to your doctor* about packing medications for diarrhoea and vomiting and use hand support if vomiting to minimise pelvic floor descent.

☑ *Travel in loose comfortable clothing.* No tight waistlines as these tend to feel uncomfortable with bloating and prolonged sitting.

☑ *On the plane, eat lightly and avoid caffeinated drinks* as they can be irritants for the bladder and may cause urinary frequency, affect your sleep and may dehydrate you.

☑ *Drink plenty of water to keep well hydrated* as this is important with prevention of DVT's.

☑ *Minimize drinking alcohol on the flight* - it is a diuretic and may cause you increased urinary frequency and may increase the risk of DVT's.

☑ *If prone to constipation with a long haul flight, then prior to flying it can be helpful to use a glycerol suppository (page 67)* either the night before or early in the morning, knowing that you have had a good evacuation of your bowels prior to flying. Using one again once you have arrived at your hotel will often make you feel more comfortable.

☑ To help prevent constipation with travelling, ensure that you *pack any fibre supplements or bowel medications and especially glycerol suppositories that you are using at home.* If you don't use fibre at home it can be helpful to take it when travelling, as your diet and fluid intake can be deficient away from home.

☑ *Try to sit properly with bladder and bowels (see pages 34 & 63)* when using the toilet although it is never easy with terminal and plane toilets.

Your own travel checklist
(Photocopy and tick it off for each trip)

Packing:
- ☐ *'Pull-along' bag* with wheels and preferably a back pack as hand luggage in the plane. If using a shoulder bag ensure it has a broad shoulder strap for carrying.
- ☐ *Pack 'light'* - Minimise heavy shoes, have mix and match clothes. Take one good coat and wear onto the plane.
- ☐ *Pack loose comfortable clothing* for plane travel. No tight waistlines.
- ☐ *Extra light cardigan* for when its cool in the plane.
- ☐ *Neck cushion* - available at the airport shops.
- ☐ *Face mask or use a loose scarf* in case someone near you has a bad cough or cold.
- ☐ *Request a travelling companion to lift all the bags* (when appropriate).
- ☐ *Read section on 'Bracing' (page 21)* before you leave. Brace before all lifting.
- ☐ *Airline travel socks* to help prevent DVTs.
- ☐ *Purse pack of flushable toilet wipes* (available in the toilet paper aisle) & also antiseptic wipes - good for wiping down public toilets to avoid hovering.
- ☐ Have a *glycerol suppository* if required *(page 67)* either the night before or early in the morning prior to flying. Take them for constipation on the holiday.
- ☐ **Talk to your doctor about the following medications -**
  - ☐ *anti-emetics* (anti vomiting).
  - ☐ *anti-diarrhoea.*
  - ☐ *anti-constipation* (fibre, osmotic laxatives such as Movicol or Osmolax).
  - ☐ *glycerol suppositories or Microlax® enemas.*
  - ☐ all usual *scripts* (and a letter from your doctor listing them).
  - ☐ *aspirin* for prevention of DVT's (discuss with doctor).

On the plane:
- ☐ *Pay attention to airline instructions* regarding prevention of deep vein thrombosis (DVT's) and do half hourly leg and ankle exercises while awake.
- ☐ *Walk* the aisles regularly.
- ☐ *Eat lightly and avoid caffeinated and alcoholic drinks.*
- ☐ *Drink water* and keep well hydrated.
- ☐ *Try to sit properly for bladder and bowels* when using the plane toilet .

When landed at your destination:
- ☐ *Use soluble fibre daily & maintain fluid intake* -can be deficient when travelling.
- ☐ *Use hand support over your perineum* (around the vagina) if vomiting.
- ☐ *Set up footstools* such as spare toilet rolls or telephone directories in your hotel room so you can evacuate your bowels easily when travelling.
- ☐ *Be aware of the local customs* regarding toilets, check with your hotel about cost and availability of toilets. Some cities have toilet maps as an app for your smart phone which can be down-loaded prior to your trip.

Chapter 15

Sexual function

Sexual dysfunction is a common yet often silent problem. It is seen in nulliparous women who are suffering pelvic pain conditions such as vulvodynia; who endure the nightmare of recurrent urinary tract infections or other chronic bladder conditions such as the Bladder Pain Syndrome (BPS and formerly known as Interstitial Cystitis).

Female sexual dysfunction can also occur in women who have pelvic floor changes following childbirth, gynaecological or colorectal surgery. Women with prolapse are often very self conscious about the change in tone and 'the look' of their vagina. They may also suffer with vaginal flatus (wind from the vagina) due to weak muscles. They are often also concerned that intercourse may worsen their prolapse (which is not true) and therefore abstain which can place pressure on relationships. It is also a common belief that once you reach menopause then libido diminishes and many women simply give up sexual intimacy which can also cause pressure on a relationship.

Initially post-operatively the doctor will usually advise you about recommencing intercourse (with penetration). Obviously due to the associated pain, discomfort and internal stiches from major gynaecological repair surgery, there can be a reluctance (often from both partners) to resume intercourse. It can be up to 8-10 weeks before the pain has disappeared allowing intercourse to happen.

It is important to use a *lubricant* initially (available at a pharmacy or online) and for post-menopausal women, using *local oestrogen (Vagifem pessaries or Ovestin cream in Australia)*, may assist with improving lubrication, decrease any pain from dryness and improve the tone and plumpness of the vaginal walls. Your specialist surgeon or GP will need to prescribe this.

Often the instructions for using local oestrogen say to start by inserting the pessaries daily for 2 weeks and then revert to inserting them twice a week. It is useful to discuss with your surgeon or GP about *commencing with twice weekly*, while this may take longer to get the desired result, it is often better tolerated by the patient. The latest advice about applying local oestrogen is to apply Ovestin cream to the anterior wall and in the lower half of the vagina and with any oestrogen cream it can be applied with your finger rather than the supplied applicator (which is often difficult to clean).

Another option if you have reservations about using local oestrogen, is to try using non-hormonal vaginal moisturisers available from pharmacies. These are available in pessary form or a gel which has as applicator and are helpful with vaginal lubrication and tissue quality. Either can be inserted twice a week into the vagina.

Since 2013, a non-surgical, non-hormonal alternative to vaginal atrophy has been available in Australia and around the world. This is a laser treatment which stimulates the body's regenerative processes to create more healthy and hydrated cells and to improve the vascularity of the vaginal mucosa. This may be a useful option much further down the track following surgery if the patient has vaginal atrophy and has had an oestrogen dependent cancer and is advised not to use local oestrogen. Discuss this with your surgeon or local GP.

Stitches used in repair surgery can be normally slow to dissolve and small pieces of suture material can discharge into the vagina for an extended period of time post-operatively. This is not a cause for concern. Any repair to the posterior wall can mean some scar-line discomfort with intercourse for a longer period of time, but this often improves quite quickly after 12 weeks.

If there is ongoing scar tissue discomfort or pain it is important to seek help. Discuss treatment options with your surgeon and you may be referred to a pelvic health physiotherapist for help. Sometimes there is a need for dilators or a therapeutic wand (see below) to be used to improve any vaginal pain, decrease persistent vaginal sensitivity or to massage tender spots or tightness in the levator muscles (the pelvic floor muscles). These muscles can develop tender areas and cause significant discomfort with intercourse for the woman.

Understanding persistent pain science will help with managing painful intercourse. Simple effective education can help women with this sometimes embarrassing topic (*Chapter 7*). There is a list of tips to improve sexual function on the following page.

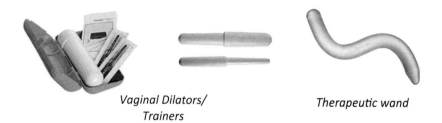

Vaginal Dilators/ Trainers   *Therapeutic wand*

Tips for improved sexual function

- Women can be quite fearful recommencing intercourse following major repair surgery, so it important to gain reassurances from your surgeon or pelvic health physiotherapist that no harm can happen and when it is safe to start intercourse again (often at 8-10 weeks).

- Work on arousal. This ensures the normal vaginal response of lubrication, engorging with blood and enlarging of the vagina will take place. If decreased libido is an issue, this can sometimes be improved by taking your time with pleasurable, physical contact (such as kissing and cuddling) and also with reading or visual material (within your comfort level).

- Take your time, don't rush things and try not to bear down with orgasm – instead tighten your pelvic floor and draw up and in and this will often improve your sexual response.

- Don't forget *'outercourse'* as well as intercourse if the pain or discomfort is too much for penetration. Ensure that there is adequate foreplay to make certain the woman is suitably aroused prior to penetration. Have the important conversation with your partner that lots of touching, embracing and kissing are important *without* always resulting in penetrative sex.

- If fully breast-feeding or post-menopausal then local oestrogen inserted in the vagina twice a week can be helpful to improve tone and lubrication of the area.

- Non-hormonal, vaginal moisturising pessaries and gels, available from the pharmacy, can also be useful if you are unable or reluctant to use local oestrogen.

- Use a lubricant: There are many different brands of lubricant available at your pharmacy. When trying a lubricant, always stop use and change it if there is stinging or irritation. Also if using condoms for contraception, think about using a non-latex condom if you have sensitivity in case there is a latex allergy.

- If there is tightness or spasm in the levator muscles (levator spasm), concentrate on relaxing your abdomen, your inner thighs and your pelvic floor and do some low, slow breathing. See *page 75*. If you contract these muscles, you will increase this spasm and tightness and make penetration more difficult. Using a vaginal dilator or wand can help with softening tender points in your pelvic floor muscles (not until 12 weeks post-operatively and with permission of your surgeon).

- Seek help early if there is ongoing pain, discomfort, decreased sensation or changes in sexual response.

16

Return to work

Following major repair surgery it is important to check with your doctor about the length of time you need to have off work. Where possible it is preferable to have six weeks off work with major gynaecological or colorectal repair surgery. Even if your job involves sitting at a computer, your perineal region (bottom) might be still quite sore and prolonged sitting may be uncomfortable. If your job involves standing, it can help to wait the six full weeks.

If you can stagger your return to work such as going back to light duties, or going back on reduced hours, this helps to build up your tolerance for work. With incontinence repairs such as a mid-urethral sling, which are often day or overnight surgery, there may be a much quicker return to work. Still be mindful of some of the guidelines.

If your job involves lifting, then it would be better to go onto light duties with no lifting until 12 weeks, to ensure adequate healing and strength of your surgery. When you consider the pain involved, the cost of surgery and the cost of having time off work with each operation, it is much more important to have the mindset that:

"Your first op, should be your best op and hopefully your last op"

Now, the surgery you are having is not like performing a service on a car. All your car services should go according to plan when following the instruction manual. When being operated on in the pelvic region, there are complex physiological structures such as the bladder and the bowel; the area is gravity dependant; the region has very fine blood vessels and nerve fibres; and there is the added complexity of varying degrees of abdominal fat pushing down. Patients may have poor tissue quality or a history of constipation or may have chronic health issues such as asthma, which means they cough regularly and forcefully.

Due to all of these factors, things don't always go according to plan like your car service will. However, I hope by following the advice in this handbook, you will feel more confident (knowledge is empowering), the outcome will be significantly improved and your understanding of this complex region will be better for life.

Your first op, should be your best op and hopefully your last op!

Chapter 17

The effects of ageing

As we age there are obvious changes that occur to muscles, collagen and the nervous system which can significantly affect bladder, bowel and pelvic floor function. Significantly though, we can hasten or exaggerate these changes, not only through bad habits, but also through inactivity and weight gain. Older people should do some form of physical exercise regardless of age, weight, health problems or abilities. While there are substantial physiological changes that do occur with ageing, one of the critical things to remember the old saying:

"If you don't use it, you will lose it".

We have already seen that if you do not maintain regular training of your pelvic floor throughout your life there will be a 5% to 10% loss of muscle strength per week which is *worse* in older age groups compared to younger age groups.[17] For pre-op and post-op, it is important to keep strengthening your pelvic floor muscles (within the restrictions provided by your surgeon) and generally to keep active and keep moving. The more sedentary you are, the more likely you are to hasten the problems that come after the age of 60 - when the ageing process really kicks in!

If you are suffering incontinence (leakage of urine, gas or faeces), it is also important to use proper incontinence pads especially when exercising as they have material in them to ensure good absorption of the urine compared with less adequate menstruation pads. Research has shown that women see urinary incontinence as a barrier to exercise (38% with moderate leakage and 85% with severe incontinence stop exercising due to UI).[73] Therefore it is better to exercise with an appropriate pad (as long as you have had your exercise regime assessed by a pelvic health physiotherapist) than to stop exercising because you are leaking. Also, if you try a device to help reduce leakage such as a pessary or *Contiform®*, remember to ask your doctor about using local supplemental oestrogen. If you cannot use an oestrogen-based product (due to previous breast cancer), try a vaginal moisturizer twice a week or a medical lubricant to help insert the devices.

As we age, fat is often deposited around the middle waist area. This increases intra-abdominal pressure, especially when exercising. Evidence tells us that if you are overweight, losing 5% to 10% of body weight can significantly help to reduce incontinence episodes and risk of worsening prolapse.[74] Finding a variety of exercises to do such as walking, dancing, cycling, swimming, Tai Chi, bowls, golf, resistance training plus many more is a prescription for a healthy life.

Dementia is another serious disease process which comes with ageing and has a detrimental effect on continence . There are many types of brain impairment that come under the broad category of dementia but almost all of them result in loss of continence control for both bladder and bowel. This often results in nursing home admission. Some recent research into continence and nursing home admission has demonstrated the staggering statistics that at 6 months after admission, 28% of nursing home residents developed urinary and faecal incontinence (dual incontinence); at 1 year 42% did so; and at 2 years, 61% had dual incontinence. Significant predictors for the length of time to developing dual incontinence were already having urinary incontinence, greater functional or cognitive deficits, more comorbidities, older age, and lesser quality of nursing home care.[75]

An important management strategy can be to institute *timed voiding* - either nursing staff prompting the client at 2 hours to go to the toilet or by the client using a watch that vibrates to alert the client to go to the toilet every two hours to help stay dry. Other neurological conditions such as Parkinson's Disease or stroke can mean the woman can suffer with slowness of their gait, leading to *functional incontinence* - where they are just too slow to get to the toilet. The impact of this will be exacerbated by any urinary or faecal urgency. See *Chapter 6* for management strategies.

Some of the changes that occur with the ageing process:

- A decline in muscle mass, although continuing to exercise regularly throughout your whole life can minimise this.
- Less elastin in the collagen which results in less strength, plasticity and elasticity of the fascia.
- Average loss of 2% per year from age 15 to 80 years in the total number of striated muscle fibres in the wall of the urethra leading to decrease in urethral closing pressure.[11]
- Stiffer smooth muscle (which is found in the bladder and internal anal sphincter).
- Urodynamic studies show advancing age is associated with a reduced bladder capacity, an increase in uninhibited contractions, decreased urinary flow rate, reduced urethral closing pressure (particularly in women), and increased postvoid residual urine volume.[76]
- Decreased number of motor neurones.
- Decreased conduction velocity of the nerves.
- Higher excitability threshold of the nerve therefore making it harder for the muscle to get going.

Chapter 18
Conclusion about change

The messages in this book are not complicated. The book contains simple, easy to implement information that will enhance your preparation for your gynaecological or colorectal repair surgery. It will help you understand what is involved in your hospital stay but, most importantly, give you strategies to look after your operation, which will hopefully transform your life.

Many women are shocked that so many habits they have adopted and had passed on from mother to daughter, are flawed and are significantly contributing to the bladder, bowel and prolapse issues they have been suffering. But they are also pleased to hear that with these simple strategies, confidence can return and self-esteem be restored.

One of the key factors in improving pelvic floor dysfunction is to be prepared to change what you have been doing in the past. Change in your behaviour, your beliefs and what are almost rituals will improve your incontinence, frequency, urgency and other bladder and bowel conditions.

"Rather than wishing for change, you first must be prepared to change."
Catherine Pulsifer

By reading this book and then contacting a pelvic health physiotherapist you will have taken the first step to a better life. You will have moved from just *wishing* for change to the next level. It might feel like you are about to climb Mt Everest, but just acknowledging you have continence issues is a big step forward.

Unless patients have heard from a friend about what is involved when they come to see a pelvic health physiotherapist, they are often surprised at the amount of education that is involved in the consultation. They may even be shocked at some of the concepts they are taught ….

Change to decaffeinated drinks? Change from hovering to urinate? Change from going 'just in case'? Change from straining to pass bowel motions? Change from being sedentary to being more active?

Initially new concepts may be difficult to accept as the bad habits have been practised for so long, but through education and putting new behaviours in place, there should be improvement in your quality of life.

"Everyone can think of the one thing that would make life better for them. But people are not so quick to answer the second question: 'What are you doing to make that change come true'."
Catherine Pulsifer

No one likes to leak urine but sometimes we want an easy path and a quick fix. Changing old bad bladder habits takes willpower, exercise, discipline, letting go of the easy old ways and doing things that, at least initially, are not familiar and comfortable. But interestingly, patients are ecstatic when their hard work starts to pay off and they can hold on longer, they are drier and they regain some sense of control with their bladder or bowel.

"Change is as inexorable as time, yet nothing meets with more resistance."
Benjamin Disraeli

How are you empowered to make these changes? Well certainly not by being ordered to do it. You now have the information, you have read the science. You are an adult and have to be the one to make the decision about the intervention. Try the decaf for a month and assess - is there improvement in the amount of leakage, the degree of urgency, the severity of your urinary frequency, the faecal incontinence? And if there is, then you make the change.

"Never stop learning, like never stop changing and growing in your life – learning helps you adapt to change more easily." **Author unknown**

Anyone can implement change - even 90 year olds - as long as you have the mindset that you can still learn new things and improve your situation. If you are fixed in your attitude, then it will be hard to inspire you. But I hope through this book I have passed on the message that what is being taught is not rocket science – but it is science-based and does involve maths (angles of how you should sit for defaecation and for emptying your bladder) and physics (counteracting forces from above, such as with cough and sneeze, with a force from below, that is, by contracting your pelvic floor muscles).

"No action, no change. Limited action, limited change. Lots of action – change occurs." **Catherine Pulsifer**

And this is the crux of all this change talk. The effort that you put in with your program will mostly be reflected in your result. The pelvic floor muscles thrive on attention even when there has been levator avulsion or nerve damage. Keep trying to maximize the potential of what is left. I hope if you get into a routine of daily pelvic floor muscle training and you implement the ideas in this book as it will make an immediate difference to your operation and more importantly contribute to its longevity. So don't delay, start today. Make the first changes and perhaps also contact your local pelvic health physiotherapist to learn how to contract your muscles correctly.

I hope this book assists you with your 'Pelvic Floor Recovery'.

Sue Croft

References

1. Deloitte Access Economics Report for The Continence Foundation of Australia 2011 *The economic impact of incontinence in Australia* https://www.continence.org.au/ data/files/Access_economics_report/dae_incontinence_report__19_april_2011.pdf

2. Neumann, P. B., Grimmer, K. A., Grant, R. E., & Gill, V. A. (2005). Physiotherapy for female stress urinary incontinence: A multicentre observational study. *Australian and New Zealand Journal of Obstetrics and Gynaecology*, 45(3), 226-232. 10.1111/ j.1479-828X.2005.00393.x

3. Sherburn M, Bird M, Carey M, Bo K, Galea M (2011) Incontinence improves in older women after intensive pelvic floor muscle training: An assessor blinded randomized controlled trial. *Neurourology and Urodynamics*, 30:317-324. doi:10.1002/.

4. Dumoulin, C., Hay-Smith, E., & Mac Habee-Seguin, G. (2014). Pelvic floor muscle training versus no treatment, or inactive control treatments, for urinary incontinence in women. *Cochrane Database of Systematic Reviews*, 5(5), CD005654. 10.1002/14651858.CD005654.pub3

5. Hagen, S., Stark, D., Maher, C., & Adams, E. (2006). Conservative management of pelvic organ prolapse in women. *Cochrane Database of Systematic Reviews* (Online), (4), CD003882. 10.1002/14651858.CD003882.pub3

6. Brubaker, L., Maher, C., Jacquetin, B., Rajamaheswari, N., von Theobald, P., & Norton, P. (2010). Surgery for pelvic organ prolapse. *Female Pelvic Medicine & Reconstructive Surgery*, 16(1), 9-19. 10.1097/SPV.0b013e3181ce959c

7. Wu, J. M., Matthews, C. A., Conover, M. M., Pate, V., & Jonsson Funk, M. (2014). Lifetime risk of stress urinary incontinence or pelvic organ prolapse surgery. *Obstetrics & Gynecology*, 123(6), 1201-1206. 10.1097/AOG.0000000000000286

8. Hagen, S., Stark, D., Glazener, C., Sinclair, L., & Ramsay, I. (2009). A randomized controlled trial of pelvic floor muscle training for stages I and II pelvic organ prolapse. International Urogynecology Journal, 20(1), 45-51. 10.1007/s00192-008-0726-4

9. Ireton, J. E., Unger, J. G., & Rohrich, R. J. (2013). The role of wound healing and its everyday application in plastic surgery: A practical perspective and systematic review. *Plastic and Reconstructive Surgery Global Open*, 1(Compendium), 1-10. 10.1097/GOX.0b013e31828ff9f4

10. Miller, J., Ashton-Miller, J., & DeLancey, J. (1998). A Pelvic Muscle Precontraction Can Reduce Cough-Related Urine Loss in Selected Women with Mild SUI. *Journal Of The American Geriatrics Society*, 46(7), 870-874. http://dx.doi.org/10.1111/j.1532-5415.1998.tb02721.x

11. Bo K, Berghmans B, Van Kampen M, Morkved S. (2007) Evidence-Based Physical Therapy for the Pelvic Floor. Bridging Science and Clinical Practice. Churchill Livingstone Elsevier.

12. Dumoulin, C., Glazener, C., & Jenkinson, D. (2011). Determining the optimal pelvic floor muscle training regimen for women with stress urinary incontinence. *Neurourology and Urodynamics*, 30(5), 746-753. 10.1002/nau.21104

13. Ferreira, M., Santos, P. C., Duarte, J. A., & Rodrigues, R. (2012). Exercise programs for women with stress urinary incontinence. *Primary Health Care* (through 2013), 22(3), 24.

14. Dietz, H. P. (2006). Pelvic floor trauma following vaginal delivery. *Current Opinion in Obstetrics and Gynecology*, 18(5), 528-537. 10.1097/01.gco.0000242956.40491.1e

15. Bø, K., Brækken, I. H., Majida, M., & Engh, M. E. (2009). Constriction of the levator hiatus during instruction of pelvic floor or transversus abdominis contraction: A 4D ultrasound study. *International Urogynecology Journal*, 20(1), 27-32. 10.1007/s00192-008-0719-3

16. Hoff Brækken, I., Majida, M., Engh, M. E., & Bø, K. (2010). Morphological changes after pelvic floor muscle training measured by 3-dimensional ultrasonography: A randomized controlled trial. *Obstetrics and Gynecology*, 115(2), 317-324. 10.1097/AOG.0b013e3181cbd35f

17. Morkved, S., & Bo, K. (2014). Effect of pelvic floor muscle training during pregnancy and after childbirth on prevention and treatment of urinary incontinence: A systematic review. *British Journal of Sports Medicine*, 48(4), 299-310. 10.1136/bjsports-2012-091758

18. Dietz, H. P., & Schierlitz, L. (2005). Pelvic floor trauma in childbirth - myth or reality? *Australian and New Zealand Journal of Obstetrics and Gynaecology*, 45(1), 3-11. 10.1111/j.1479-828X.2005.00363.x

19. Dietz, & Simpson. (2008). Levator trauma is associated with pelvic organ prolapse. BJOG: *An International Journal of Obstetrics & Gynaecology*, 115(8), 979-984. 10.1111/j.1471-0528.2008.01751.x

20. Dietz, H. P. (2009). Pelvic Floor Assessment. *Fetal and Maternal Medicine Review*, 20(1), 49-66. 10.1017/S096553950900237X

21. Dietz, H. P. (2013). Pelvic floor trauma in childbirth. *Australian and New Zealand Journal of Obstetrics and Gynaecology*, 53(3), 220-230. 10.1111/ajo.12059

22. Thompson J, O'Sullivan P, Briffa NK and Neumann P (2007). Comparison of transperineal and transabdominal ultrasound in the assessment of voluntary pelvic floor muscle contractions and functional manoeuvres in continent and incontinent women. *International Urogynaecology Journal*, Volume 18, Number 7, Pages 779-786.

23. http://merriam-webster.com/dictionary/brace;http://www.thefreedictionary.com/bracing [Accessed 13 Nov. 2017].

24. O'Sullivan P, Caneiro JP, O'Keefe M, O'Sullivan K (2016) Unravelling the complexity of low back pain *J Orthop Sports Phys Ther* 2016; 46(11); 932-937

25. Sapsford R, Richardson C, Stanton W, (2006) Sitting posture affects pelvic floor muscle activity in parous women: An observational study. *Australian Journal of Physiotherapy* 219-222.

26. Sinaki M, Itoi E, Wahner HW, Wollan P, Gelzcer R, Mullan BP, et al. Stronger back muscles reduce the incidence of vertebral fractures: a prospective 10 year follow-up of postmenopausal women. *Bone.* 2002;30(6):836-41.

27. Gerten, K. (2008). Intraabdominal pressure changes associated with lifting: Implications for postoperative activity restrictions. *Am J Obstet Gynecol*, 198(3), 306.e1-306.e5. 10.1016/j.ajog.2007.09.004

28. Yamasato K, Oyama I, Kaneshiro B (2014)Intra-abdominal Pressure with Pelvic Floor Dysfunction. *Journal of Reproductive Medicine* 409-413 2014

29. International Continence Society Terminology page *(https://www.ics.org/terminology/5)* [Accessed 15 Dec. 2017].

30. Zhong YH, Fang Y, Zhou JZ, Tang Y, Gong SM, Ding XQ. Effectiveness and Safety of Patient initiated Single-dose versus Continuous Low-dose Antibiotic Prophylaxis for Recurrent Urinary Tract Infections in Postmenopausal Women: a Randomized Controlled Study. *J Int Med Res*. 2011. 39(6):2335-43

31. Infectious Diseases Society of America. (2017, October 5). Women who get frequent UTIs may reduce risk by drinking plenty of water. ScienceDaily. Retrieved February8,2018from www.sciencedaily.com/releases/2017/10/171005190252.htm

32. Jepson R, Williams G, Craig J (2012) Cranberries for preventing urinary tract infections. *Cochrane Database System Review* Oct 17; 10: CD001321.

33. Terris, M. K., Issa, M. M., & Tacker, J. R. (2001). Dietary supplementation with cranberry concentrate tablets may increase the risk of nephrolithiasis. *Urology*, 57(1), 26-29. 10.1016/S0090-4295(00)00884-0

34. Abrams P, Cardozo L, Wagg A. 2016 *Incontinence* 6th Edition 2017, Volume 2 page 1525.

35. Bergman, A., Sih, A. and Weiss, J. (2015). Nocturia: an overview of evaluation and treatment. *Bladder*, 2(2), p.13.

36. Weiss JP, Weinberg AC, Blaivas JG (2008) New aspects of the classification of nocturia. *Curr Urol Rep* 9: 362-367.

37. Dietz, H. P., Chantarasorn, V. and Shek, K. L. (2010), Levator avulsion is a risk factor for cystocele recurrence. *Ultrasound Obstet Gynecol*, 36: 76–80. doi:10.1002/uog.7678

38. Wong M, Harmanali O, Mehmet A, Dandolu V, Grody M (2003) Collagen content of non support tissue in pelvic organ prolapse and stress urinary incontinence. *American Journal of Obstetrics & Gynaecology* Volume 189, Issue 6 , Pages 1597-1599, December 2003.http://www.ajog.org/article/S0002-9378(03)01192-X/abstract.

39. Vierhout M, Terlouw E (2001) My mother has a prolapse: will I get one? *International Urogynaecology Journal*, 12 (supplement3), abstract 231, p 142.

40. Castori, M. (2012).Ehlers-danlos syndrome, hypermobility type: An underdiagnosed hereditary connective tissue disorder with mucocutaneous, articular, and systemic manifestations. *ISRN Dermatology*, 2012, 1-22. 10.5402/2012/751768

41. Jarrett, M. E., Wijffels, N. A., Slater, A., Cunningham, C., & Lindsey, I. (2010;2009;). Enterocoele is a marker of severe pelvic floor weakness. Colorectal Disease : *The Official Journal of the Association of Coloproctology of Great Britain and Ireland,* 12(7), e158-162. 10.1111/j.1463-1318.2009.02024.x

42. Miedel, A., Ek, M., Tegerstedt, G., Mæhle-Schmidt, M., Nyrén, O., & Hammarström, M. (2011). Short-term natural history in women with symptoms indicative of pelvic organ prolapse. *International Urogynecology Journal, 22(4)*, 461-468. 10.1007/s00192-010-1305-z

43. Hagen S, Stark D, Glazener C, Dickson S, Barry S, Elders A (2014) POPPY Trial Collaborators. Individualized pelvic floor muscle training in women with pelvic organ prolapse (POPPY): A multi-centre randomized controlled trial. *Lancet, 383(9919)*, 796-806. 10.1016/S0140-6736(13)61977-7

44. Goh J, Flynn M (2017) *Obstetrics and Gynaecology Examination* 4th Edition Elsevier Australia, Chatswood, NSW.

45. Yong C, Al-Salihi S, Carey M. Laparoscopic and robotic sacrocervicopexy with subtotal hysterectomy for management of uterine prolapse *Neurourology and Urodynamics* July 2017 ICS abstract, Volume 36, Supplement 3, abstract 436

46. Schlichte, M. J., & Guidry, J. (2015). Current cervical carcinoma screening guidelines. Journal of *Clinical Medicine, 4(5)*, 918-932. 10.3390/jcm4050918

47. Birmingham Bowel Clinic. (n.d.). Anorectal Physiology Tests | Birmingham Bowel Clinic. [online] Available at: http://www.birminghambowelclinic.co.uk/investigations/anorectal-physiology-tests/ [Accessed 15 Jan. 2018].

48. Rieger, N., Tjandra, J., & Solomon, M. (2004). Endoanal and endorectal ultrasound: Applications in colorectal surgery. *ANZ Journal of Surgery, 74(8)*, 671-675. 10.1111/j.1445-1433.2004.02884.x

49. Markwell S, Sapsford R (1995) Physiotherapy management of obstructed defaecation. *Australian Journal of Physiotherapy*; 41:279–83.

50. The Heart Foundation. (n.d.). Fruit and vegetables. [online] Available at: https://www.heartfoundation.org.au/healthy-eating/food-and-nutrition/fruit-and-vegetables [Accessed 2 Feb. 2018].

51. Bell,J Bolin T, Cowan A, Korman M, Kamm M, Lemberg D, Ledder O, Day A, Leong R, Collings K (2015) *Constipation and Bloating,* produced by the Gut Foundation.

52. Heaton K, LewisS (1997) Stool form as a useful guide to intestinal transit time. *Scandinavian Journal of Gastroenterology.* Vol32, No 9, pp 920-924

53. McClurg D, Walker K, Aitchison P, Jamieson K, Dickinson L, Paul L, Cunnington A (2016). Abdominal massage for the relief of constipation in people with Parkinson's: A qualitative study. *Parkinsons Disease*, 201610.1155/2016/4842090

54. Labat, J., Riant, T., Robert, R., Amarenco, G., Lefaucheur, J., & Rigaud, J. (2008). Diagnostic criteria for pudendal neuralgia by pudendal nerve entrapment (nantes criteria). *Neurourology and Urodynamics, 27(4)*, 306-310. 10.1002/nau.20505

55. https://www.glowm.com/section_view/heading/Pudendal%20Neuralgia/item/691#27971) [accessed 3 Jan 2018].

56. Moseley G., & Butler D. (2017). *Explain Pain Supercharged* (1st ed., p. 244 pages). Adelaide, Australia: Noigroup Publications.

57. Moseley G, & Butler, D(2013). *Explain Pain* Adelaide, Australia: Noigroup Publications.

58. Grace, P, Strand, K., Galer E., Urban, D., Wang, X., Baratta, M, Watkins, L. (2016). Morphine paradoxically prolongs neuropathic pain in rats by amplifying spinal NLRP3 inflammasome activation. *Proceedings of the National Academy of Sciences of the United States of America, 113(24)*, E3441-E3450. 10.1073/pnas.1602070113

59. Yasmato K, Oyama I, Kaneshiro B (2014) Intraabdominal pressure with pelvic floor dysfunction. Do postoperative restrictions make sense? Journal of Reproductive Medicine Vol59, Number 7

60. Nygaard, I. E., Hamad, N. M., & Shaw, J. M. (2013). Activity restrictions after gynecologic surgery: Is there evidence? *International Urogynecology Journal*, 24(5), 719-724. 10.1007/s00192-012-2026-2

61. Vonk Noordegraaf, A., Huirne, J. A. F., Brölmann, H. A. M., Mechelen, v., W, & Anema, J. R. (2011). Multidisciplinary convalescence recommendations after gynaecological surgery: A modified delphi method among experts. *Gynaecology*, 118 (13), 1557-1567. 10.1111/j.1471-0528.2011.03091.x

124

62. O'Dell, K. K., Morse, A. N., Crawford, S. L., & Howard, A. (2007). Vaginal pressure during lifting, floor exercises, jogging, and use of hydraulic exercise machines. *International Urogynecology Journal*, 18(12), 1481-1489. 10.1007/s00192-007-0387-8

63. Coleman, T. J., Hamad, N. M., Shaw, J. M., Egger, M. J., Hsu, Y., Hitchcock, R., . . . Nygaard, I. E. (2015;2014;). Effects of walking speeds and carrying techniques on intra-abdominal pressure in women. *International Urogynecology Journal*, 26(7), 967-974. 10.1007/s00192-014-2593-5

64. Mueller, M. G., Lewicky-Gaupp, C., Collins, S. A., Abernethy, M. G., Alverdy, A., & Kenton, K. (2017). Activity restriction recommendations and outcomes after reconstructive pelvic surgery: A randomized controlled trial. *Obstetrical & Gynecological Survey*, 72(7), 410-424. 10.1097/OGX.0000000000000462

65. Shin, E. J. (2011). Surgical Treatment of Rectal Prolapse. *Journal of the Korean Society of Coloproctology*, 27(1), 5–12. http://doi.org/10.3393/jksc.2011.27.1.5

66. Maher, C. M., Feiner, B., Baessler, K., & Glazener, C. M. A. (2011). Surgical management of pelvic organ prolapse in women: The updated summary version cochrane review. *International Urogynecology Journal*, 22(11), 1445-1457. 10.1007/s00192-011-1542-9

67. Vakili, B., Zheng, Y. T., Loesch, H., Echols, K. T., Franco, N., & Chesson, R. R. (2005). Levator contraction strength and genital hiatus as risk factors for recurrent pelvic organ prolapse. Am J Obstet Gynecol, 192(5), 1592-1598. doi:10.1016/j.ajog.2004.11.022

68. Rodrigo, N., Wong, V., Shek, K. L., Martin, A., & Dietz, H. P. (2014). The use of 3-dimensional ultrasound of the pelvic floor to predict recurrence risk after pelvic reconstructive surgery. *Australian and New Zealand Journal of Obstetrics and Gynaecology,* 54(3), 206-211. 10.1111/ajo.12171

69. Dietz, H. P., Hankins, K. J., & Wong, V. (2014). The natural history of cystocele recurrence. *International Urogynecology Journal*, 25(8), 1053-1057. 10.1007/s00192-014-2339-4

70. Vergeldt, T. F. M., Weemhoff, M., IntHout, J., & Kluivers, K. B. (2015). Risk factors for pelvic organ prolapse and its recurrence: a systematic review. *International Urogynecology Journal*, 26(11), 1559–1573. http://doi.org/10.1007/s00192-015-2695-8

71. https://www.cdc.gov/physicalactivity/basics/adults/index.htm [Accessed18Feb. 2018]

72. Serra, A., Lemes, B., Silva, J., Bocalini, D., Suzuk, F., Albertini, R., Caetano, A., Carvalho, P., Arsa, G. and Vieira, S. (2013). Different land-based exercise training programs to improve bone health in postmenopausal women. *Medical Science and Technology*, [online] 54, pp.158-163. Available at: https://www.medscitechnol.com/download/index/idArt/889899 [Accessed 20 Feb. 2018].

73. Nygaard I, Girts T, Fultz N, Kinchen K, Pohl G, Sternfeld B. (2005) Is urinary incontinence a barrier to exercise in women? Obstetrics & Gynaecology Vol 106 (Issue 2)

74. Wing RR, Creasman JM, West DS, et al. Improving urinary incontinence in overweight and obese women through modest weight loss. Obstet Gynecol. 2010;116(2 Pt 1):284–92

75. Bliss DZ, Gurvich OV, Eberly LE, Harms S. Time to and predictors of dual incontinence in older nursing home admissions. Neurourology and Urodynamics. 2018;37:229–236. https://doi.org/10.1002/nau.23279

76. Siroky, M. B. (2004). The aging bladder. *Reviews in Urology*, 6 Suppl 1(Suppl 1), S3-S7.

Appendix 1: Useful books and links

BOOKS

'Pelvic Floor Essentials'
by Sue Croft (2018)
Essential pelvic floor information for those before or following childbirth and not undergoing gynaecological or colorectal repair surgery.
'Constipation and Bloating : An information booklet'
The Gut Foundation (2015).
A very thorough guide on the bowel.
'Explain Pain' and **'Explain Pain Supercharged'** (2013, 2017)
Excellent texts on understanding persistent pain by David Butler and Lorimer Moseley. Noigroup Publications, Adelaide.
'The Protectometer' (2015)
A patient-directed work book to help the patients with persistent pain by David Butler and Lorimer Moseley, Noigroup Publications, Adelaide.

WEBSITES

http://suecroftphysiotherapistblog.wordpress.com/
Blogs (articles) related to pelvic floor dysfunction written by Sue Croft.
http://www.continence.org.au/.
Phone number: 1800 33 00 66
The Continence Foundation of Australia is the peak body dealing with incontinence whose charter is education & dissemination of education material such as leaflets & books on all matters related to continence. Many of the brochures are in multiple languages.
http://www.pelvicfloorexercise.com.au/
Pelvic Floor Exercise Online Shop for all your pelvic health products.
https://www.birthtrauma.org.au/
ABTA - Australasian Birth Trauma Association. A support association for women who have suffered a traumatic birth.
http://www.bladderbowel.gov.au/
This is a very informative Australian Government website covering information about the bladder and bowel.
http://www.physiotherapy.asn.au/APAWCM/controls/findaphysio.asps
This is the link to the *'Find a Physio'* site of the Australian Physiotherapy Association. Enter 'Continence and women's health' and your state and all the listings for physiotherapists who work in this specialised area will be shown. You can then choose the most convenient.
http://www.daa.asn.au/
The site to locate a dietician near you to help with more complex management of FODMAPS, IBS, fibre intake, constipation and bloating.
www.hada.org.au, Donations, Africa-Medical Training, AFR-010 HADA
If you would like to donate to the fistula and prolapse repair work that Dr Hannah Krause and Professor Judith Goh perform in Africa. 100% of the money raised goes to their work.

Appendix 2 : Example bladder diary

24 to 48 HOUR FLUID INPUT / OUTPUT CHART

Starting date / /

Degree of urge:
0 = no urge ++ = moderate urge
+ = slight urge +++ = busting

OUTPUT (wees—normal volumes 350 to 500mls)

Time	Amount (mls)	Leakage	Triggers	Degree of Urge
6.10 am	340	Small amount urge	Full bladder	+ + +
7.30am	100	Nil	Going out	
9.30am	200	Large amount urge	Queue in toilet	
11.00am	Small amount	Small amount	Sneeze	
12.30pm		Nil	Bowels opened	
1.30pm	70	Nil	Going to appointment	
4.30pm	240	Medium amount	Busting	
5.10pm	70	Nil	Leaving work	O
7.10pm	100	Nil		+
9.30pm	200	Nil		
10.00pm	30	Nil	Before bed	
2.00am	200	Large amount urge	Woke me	+ + +
7.00am	250mls	Nil	Waking	+ + +

INPUT (drinks)

Time	Amount (mls)	Type
6.30am	100	Orange Juice
	200	Decaf coffee
9.30am	200	Water
10.30am	200	Coffee
12 noon	200	Juice
	200	Decaf Tea
3.00pm	200	Coffee
4.00pm	200	Water
5.45pm	100	Scotch and dry
6.30pm	100	Water
7.00pm	200	Coffee
10.00pm	100	Water with medication

- This can be done at any time. Try to do one every birthday.
- Do not necessarily try to repeat a normal day, try to implement the changes discussed in the book.
- Make sure to complete the form on a day you are mostly at home.
- Find a large container and place in toilet bowl. Wee into this then pour into a measuring jug and measure in milliliters and not fluid ounces.
- Then record each void (wee).
- Also record everything you drink in the 'Input' section.
- Complete the form over a 24 hour period. It is helpful to continue measurements for 48 hours if possible.

24 to 48 HOUR FLUID INPUT / OUTPUT CHART

Starting date / /

Degree of urge:
0 = no urge ++ = moderate urge
+ = slight urge +++ = busting

OUTPUT (wees—normal volumes 350 to 500mls)

Time	Amount	Leakage	Triggers	Degree of Urge

INPUT (drinks)

Time	Amount	Type

- *This can be done at any time. Try to do one every birthday.*
- *Do not necessarily try to repeat a normal day, try to implement the changes discussed in the book.*
- *Make sure to complete the form on a day you are mostly at home.*
- *Find a large container and place in toilet bowl. Wee into this then pour into a measuring jug and measure in milliliters and not fluid ounces.*
- *Then record each void (wee).*
- *Also record everything you drink in the 'Input' section.*
- *Complete the form over a 24 hour period. It is helpful to continue measurements for 48 hours if possible.*

BOWEL DIARY

Starting date: / /

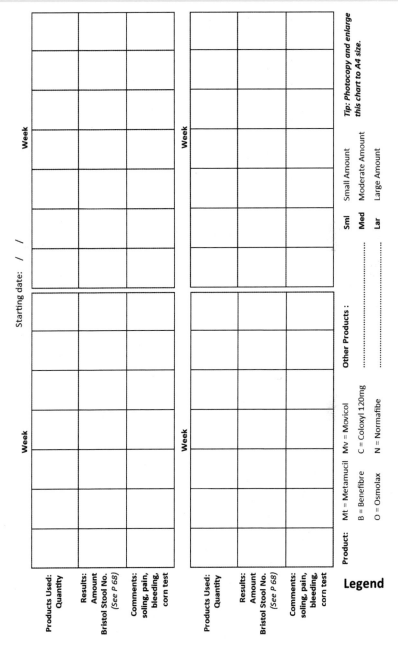

Week

Week

Week

Week

| Products Used: Quantity |
| Results: Amount |
| Bristol Stool No. *(See P 68)* |
| Comments: soling, pain, bleeding, corn test |

| Products Used: Quantity |
| Results: Amount |
| Bristol Stool No. *(See P 68)* |
| Comments: soling, pain, bleeding, corn test |

Legend

Product:	Mt = Metamucil	Mv = Movicol	**Other Products :**	**Sml**	Small Amount	**Tip:** *Photocopy and enlarge this chart to A4 size.*
	B = Benefibre	C = Coloxyl 120mg	....	**Med**	Moderate Amount	
	O = Osmolax	N = Normafibe	....	**Lar**	Large Amount	

129

Pelvic Floor Essentials

Many women suffer with pelvic floor dysfunction such as stress urinary incontinence and prolapse following vaginal deliveries. Others have bladder issues such as an overactive bladder or recurrent urinary tract infections without having had children at all. Following the success of my first book *Pelvic Floor Recovery - Physiotherapy for Gynaecological and Colorectal Surgery*, I have written this second book, **'Essentials',** to assist women in learning how to correct any bladder and pelvic floor problems using conservative measures whether having had children or not. This book includes information such as:

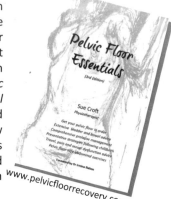

www.pelvicfloorrecovery.com

- *Correct activation of the pelvic floor and abdominal muscles.*
- *Pelvic floor muscle training program.*
- *Good bladder and bowel habits and effective toilet positioning.*
- *Conservative prolapse management strategies.*
- *'Pelvic floor friendly' abdominal exercises.*
- *Relaxation, breath awareness and persistent pain education.*
- *Sport, sexual function and travel advice.*

The book is easy to read and has simple, clear diagrams and illustrations to demonstrate the anatomy and exercises. It is small enough to sit on your bedside table for regular review and to help your pelvic floor stay in good shape forever.

"This book brings together all the essential factors of bladder control, fluid management and bowel function, including prolapse prevention and sexual function in a way that is clear with a focused approach to the problems women experience. Like her first book, Sue has included practical advice and tips in highlighted sections making this a very easy read for all women as well as a useful resource for clinicians."

Dr Irmina Nahon, PhD.
Assistant Professor in Physiotherapy, University of Canberra.